SO-DYE-282

Children's Medications:

A Parent's Guide

RICHARD D. BATES, PHARMD

Assistant Professor of
Pharmacy Practice and Pediatric Pharmacy
College of Pharmacy
Washington State University
Spokane, Washington
Formerly
Fellow in Pediatric Pharmacotherapy
College of Pharmacy
The Ohio State University
and Children's Hospital
Columbus, Ohio

and

MILAP C. NAHATA, PHARMD

Professor of Pharmacy and Pediatrics
Colleges of Pharmacy and Medicine
The Ohio State University
and Children's Hospital
Columbus, Ohio

Harvey Whitney Books • Cincinnati, Ohio • 1996

Library of Congress Cataloging-in-Publication Data

Bates, Richard D., 1968–
    Children's medications: a parent's guide / Richard D. Bates and
Milap C. Nahata.
        p.   cm.
    Includes bibliographical references and index.
    ISBN 0–929375–16–5
    1. Pediatric pharmacology—Popular works.   I. Nahata, Milap C.
II. Title.
    RJ560.B385   1995   95–8561
    615'.1'083—dc20   CIP

All rights reserved. Reproduction or translation of any part of this work beyond
that permitted by Sections 107 or 108 of the 1976 United States Copyright Act
without permission of the copyright owner is unlawful. No part of this publication
may be utilized by any information storage and retrieval system, or transmitted, in
any form or by any means, electronic, mechanical, photocopying, recording, or otherwise, without prior written permission from the publisher.

NOTICE: The authors and publisher have made every effort to provide
accurate information in this book. Due to periodic changes in information, and the possibility of errors, readers are advised to consult
an appropriate physician or pharmacist when any doubt exists. The
authors and Harvey Whitney Books Company disclaim all liability in
connection with the use of the information provided herein.

Copyright 1996 by Harvey Whitney Books Company

4906 Cooper Road, P.O. Box 42696 • Cincinnati, Ohio 45242

Printed on acid-free paper in the United States of America

PREFACE

We recognized the need for this book while we were preparing the book entitled *Children's Medications: A Guide for Schools and Day Care Centers.* When reviewing the textbooks and references we used to write that book, we noticed that there was a lack of one clear, concise book written for parents with little or no background in a healthcare field. Even though there are numerous books on medications written for non-health professionals, each one lacked something important: information on the use of medications in infants, children, and adolescents. Also, information about medicine storage, medication interactions, and adverse side effects was either incomplete or difficult to read.

We have written *Children's Medications: A Parent's Guide* to achieve two objectives. First, to not only describe what each medicine is for, but also to furnish information on the correct doses, other medications it may interact with, adverse side effects, the correct way to store and give the medicine, and special warnings related to each one. Second, to prepare a book on medications that is unique in its focus on infants, children, and adolescents. Additional information is provided on the use of many of these drugs in adults. All of this is presented in clear, easy-to-understand language.

A conference on medication errors was attended by members of the American Medical Association, the American Nurses Association, and the American Society of Health-System Pharmacists. All participants agreed that the patients and families are an important part of the healthcare team. We hope that *A Parent's Guide* will help parents become an active part of this team by keeping them informed about the medicines they are giving to their children. If this book helps prevent one medicine-related injury, or answers someone's question on how to correctly give a medicine, we will have accomplished our objectives. We encourage you to contact us with your comments or suggestions.

RICHARD D. BATES, PHARMD
MILAP C. NAHATA, PHARMD

Columbus, Ohio • July, 1995

TABLE OF CONTENTS

ACKNOWLEDGMENTS

The assistance of Timothy Welty, PharmD, and the editorial staff at Harvey Whitney Books Company is appreciated. In particular, the patience and hard work of Donna Thordsen, RN, BA, who reviewed the numerous revisions of this book and made useful suggestions, are greatly appreciated.

We wish to thank Jeff Chu, Hue Ong, and Romando Cruz for preparing the art work.

We are grateful to our wives, Nancy and Suchitra, for their editing, patience, and support throughout the development and writing of this book. This is dedicated to them.

INTRODUCTION

Not too long ago people would have questioned the need for a medication book focused on children. They would have stated that children are small adults, and therefore, should be given half or part of the adult dose. Recent research has shown that children not only differ from adults in how their bodies handle drugs, but also from one another at different ages.

What are children and how do they differ from each other and adults? In this publication, the term "children" refers to various age groups: neonate (birth to 1 month old), infant (1 to 12 months old), child (1 to 12 years old), and adolescent (12 to 17 years old). As children grow into adults, a variety of changes occurs that affect how a medicine is digested, stored in the body, and removed from the body. These changes occur continuously as children grow and develop. This is why the dose of a medicine given to an 8-month-old infant is different than the dose used for a 10-year-old child.

Even though these changes are known, little research is performed to help us understand how they affect the safety and efficacy of medicine given to children. Many medications given to children have not been approved by the Food and Drug Administration for use in children. However, when a child has a chronic disease (such as cystic fibrosis, heart murmurs, or a seizure disorder), healthcare professionals cannot wait for completion of the necessary research before approval is obtained. Therefore, many of the doses given are not based on extensive research, but on the experience health professionals have had with the medicine in treating children.

Many people are doing their best to make medication use in children as safe as possible, but more research is still needed. Research is needed in order to completely understand how the body affects medications and how medications affect the body in this age group. Through this research appropriate doses, cautions, and adverse side effects that are age specific can be found. Until then, health professionals, parents, and teachers must remember that what is best for the adult may not be best for the child.

This book reflects information from many different sources that has been gathered, examined, and combined to provide a complete picture of many different medicines. The material then was translated from the hard-to-read medical terminology into an easy-to-read language.

The information is presented in detailed medication charts that cover everything from what the medicine does and how it works to special precautions that must be taken while the child is receiving this medicine. In addition, we have added several sections that are not routinely found in medication books. These sections are:

MEDICATION STORAGE gives advice on how to store medicine at home. It also tells how to handle a call to 911 or the Poison Control Center if an accident does occur.

MEDICATION ADMINISTRATION THE CORRECT WAY outlines step-by-step how to give the medicine if no instructions have been given to you by a physician, nurse, or pharmacist.

CALCULATION OF MEDICATION DOSES shows how to calculate the appropriate dose of a medicine by easy examples.

We believe we have accomplished what we set out to do—provide a user friendly medication book that goes beyond simply listing medications and the problems associated with them. This book answers questions about how to administer medicines correctly, and most importantly, how to prevent problems from occurring while they are being used.

MEDICATION STORAGE

What is the ideal place for storing medicine? Several factors are important to consider.

First, and most important, **keep *all* medicine out of the reach of children.** Children are extremely curious, not only as infants, but also when they get older. The curiosity of children should never be underestimated, whatever their age. Poison Control Centers frequently receive calls regarding children of all ages who, for no apparent reason, have swallowed a potentially lethal substance.

All medicines should be kept in a place that is very inaccessible to children, whether this means placing them on the top shelf of a child-proof cabinet or in a locked safe. Do not expect a child-proof container to prevent the child from getting the medicine. A child-proof container is one that only takes longer for a young child to open than an adult.

If the medicine is kept in a locked cabinet that is accessible to children, be sure the cabinet is always locked, whether or not you are in the room. If the cabinet is not locked when you are in the room, it is no better than placing the medicine on the floor in front of the child. It may take less than a minute for a child to get the medicine and take enough to cause serious harm.

What about medicine that needs to be refrigerated? It is impractical to lock a refrigerator. However, some basic steps can be taken to decrease the chance of the child getting into the medicine. The easiest is to put the medicine on the top shelf of the refrigerator. If the child can reach or get to the top shelf, the medicine can be hidden behind something on that shelf. The medicine then will be out of the child's sight and, hopefully, out of mind. If you believe it is necessary to make it more difficult for the child to open the refrigerator, velcro straps that can be attached to the door are available. However, this provides only limited protection.

Second, moisture and direct sunlight may damage some medicines, making them less effective. Unless otherwise directed, medicine always should be kept in a cool, dry place away from sunlight.

Third, always keep the medicine in the original container it was dispensed in from the pharmacy. It is required by law that all medicine dispensed from the pharmacy be placed in child-proof containers unless the patient specifies otherwise. As mentioned earlier, a child-proof container is not a guarantee that a child cannot open it. It only means that it usually takes young children longer to open it than an adult. It is this extra time that may allow you to stop the child from getting hurt.

Even with all the care you take in storing medicines, you may still find young children with an open bottle. If this occurs, you *must* do the following:

1) **Remain calm.** If you panic, that does not help the child and may even delay the administration of the proper treatment that may save the child's life.

2) **Take the medicine container and medicine away from the child, but keep the container near you.**

3) **Do not let the child leave your sight.** Some medicine may cause the child to become dizzy and fall or pass out. It is best that he remains near you, sitting or lying on the floor. If he refuses, do not waste time trying to get him to sit or lie on the floor, but at least keep him in your sight.

4) **Call 911 or the Poison Control Center before you do anything else.** Never try to make the child vomit unless otherwise directed to do so by a specially trained health professional. Keep the Poison Control Center's number readily available.

5) **When talking to 911 or the Poison Control Center, remain calm and give them all the information requested.** Some of the questions they ask may seem unnecessary to you, but it is necessary to determine if the child has been poisoned or not.

Emergency Numbers

Poison Control Center
Telephone: _____

Hospital Emergency Room
Telephone: _____

Hospital Emergency Room
Telephone: _____

Physician
Telephone: _____

MEDICATION ADMINISTRATION: THE CORRECT WAY

Today, medicine comes in a variety of dosage forms. A dosage form is the form the medicine comes in, such as capsule, tablet, liquid. Listed below are a variety of different dosage forms. Under each one, detailed instructions are provided on how to administer it correctly. If at any time you have difficulty understanding the directions for administering the medicine call the child's physician or a pharmacist for help.

ORAL

Liquids

Liquid medications are probably the most convenient and easy way to give medicine to infants and young children. When giving a liquid medicine, never use an ordinary kitchen teaspoon or tablespoon. Kitchen utensils usually do not deliver the correct volume of liquid; therefore, underdosage or overdosage may occur. Always use a dropper, spoon, syringe, or measuring cup manufactured specifically for giving medicine. This is the only way to be sure that the correct dose is given. These usually are marked so as little as one-fourth, or less, of a teaspoon of liquid can be given accurately.

One problem when using these devices is how to get the medicine into them without making a mess. It may be difficult, unless you have been shown the proper way. The following steps should make it easier for you to administer liquid medicine.

Oral Medication Syringe

There are basically two proper ways to put the correct amount of medicine into the syringe.

1) The easiest is to pour a small volume of the liquid medicine into a medicine cup, or any other small cup you have. Put the tip of the syringe into the liquid in the cup and pull back on the plunger to withdraw the proper volume of liquid. Make sure that the tip of the syringe remains under the top level of the liquid so air is not drawn into the syringe. The remaining liquid should then be poured back into the medicine bottle.

2) Another method, which may take some practice, is to use a syringe adapter. This is a triangular shaped plastic device. The medicine

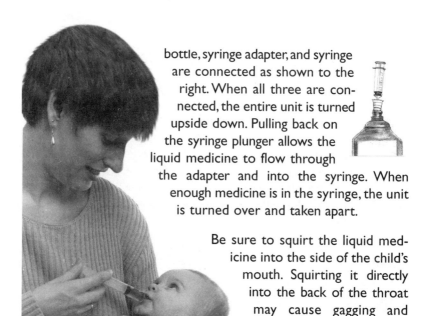

bottle, syringe adapter, and syringe are connected as shown to the right. When all three are connected, the entire unit is turned upside down. Pulling back on the syringe plunger allows the liquid medicine to flow through the adapter and into the syringe. When enough medicine is in the syringe, the unit is turned over and taken apart.

Be sure to squirt the liquid medicine into the side of the child's mouth. Squirting it directly into the back of the throat may cause gagging and coughing. Squirt the liquid slowly enough to allow the child to swallow naturally.

The syringe should be rinsed with warm water after each use.

Oral Medicine Dropper

The dropper is usually part of the medicine bottle you receive from the pharmacy. When a dose is needed simply withdraw the correct volume into the dropper.

Be sure to drop the liquid into the side of the mouth to avoid possible gagging and coughing.

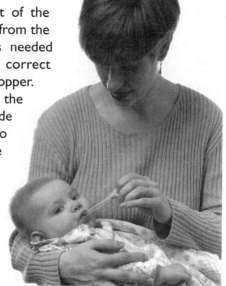

The dropper should be rinsed with warm water if it is not a part of the medicine bottle.

Medicine Spoon

The easiest way to get liquid medicine into a medicine spoon is to hold the spoon upright. With the spoon upright, and using the markings on the side as guides, pour the correct volume of medicine into the spoon. Before giving the medicine, you may want to tell the child to pretend she is drinking a glass of milk or juice. Put the spoon up to her lips and tilt it. The liquid should flow into the child's mouth slowly enough to allow normal swallowing.

The spoon should be rinsed with warm water after each use.

One problem that occasionally arises when trying to administer liquid medicine to a child is that it tastes bad. Some medicines taste relatively good, like amoxicillin; others taste bad, like prednisolone. When a child finds that a liquid medicine tastes bad, she may not want to take any liquid medicine, especially any that look like the original one.

A way to overcome this is by mixing the medicine in a small volume of water or fruit juice. This will help mask the taste of the medicine so the child can take it. If this is done, the child must drink the entire mixture to be sure the whole dose was taken. However, not all liquid medicine should be diluted in water or fruit juice. Contact the child's physician or a pharmacist for guidance.

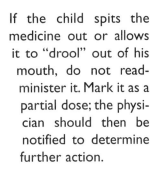

If the child spits the medicine out or allows it to "drool" out of his mouth, do not readminister it. Mark it as a partial dose; the physician should then be notified to determine further action.

Tablets and Capsules

Tablets and capsules are usually the easiest and cleanest way to give medicine to older children. As a rule, unless otherwise instructed by a physician or pharmacist, they should always be swallowed whole with water. This is because some tablets and capsules have protective properties that may either protect the stomach from becoming upset or the medicine from being harmed by the acid in the stomach. Others may have long-acting properties that allow the medicine to be given one or two times a day. If these tablets and capsules are chewed, cut, crushed, or opened, the protective and/or long-acting properties may be destroyed and the drug then could possibly harm the child. To be sure the correct amount of medicine is being given in the safest way, tablets and capsules should **not** be crushed, chewed, cut, or opened unless otherwise instructed by a physician or pharmacist.

When a certain medicine is not manufactured in a liquid form, a tablet or capsule is prescribed. This is a problem for infants or young children, since they are unable to swallow a tablet or capsule. Many tablets or capsules can be changed into liquid medicine by the pharmacist at the pharmacy. Others do not have to be converted to liquid medicine, because the tablet or capsule can be mixed with liquid or food at home. To do this, just crush the tablet or open the capsule and sprinkle the powder into a small volume of water or fruit juice or over a small amount of ice cream or soft food. To be sure the entire dose is taken, the child must drink or eat the entire mixture. Mixing medicine with food or liquid should be done only under the direction of a physician or pharmacist.

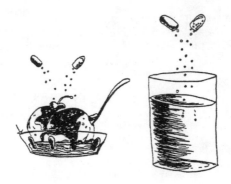

OTIC (Ear)

A. Wash your hands before giving the medicine.

B. Warm the medicine to **body temperature** by holding the bottle between your hands for several minutes.

C. Place the child on his side so the affected ear is easily accessible.

D. If ear drainage is present, gently clean the ear canal with a cotton swab.

E. Straighten the ear canal by the following methods:

   Child younger than 3 years: hold the ear lobe and pull down and back.

   Child older than 3 years: hold the upper part of the ear and pull up and back.

F. Without touching the dropper to the ear, drop the prescribed number of drops into the ear. It is best if the drops are placed onto the side of the ear canal and not dropped directly down the ear canal.

G. Have the child remain on his side for about 5 minutes.

H. If the other ear requires drops, repeat steps C to G.

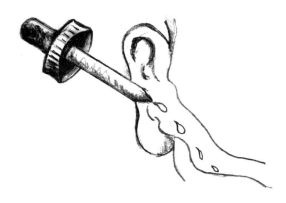

OPHTHALMIC (Eye)

Drops

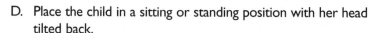

A. Wash your hands before giving the medicine.

B. Warm the medicine to **room temperature**.

C. Clean all secretions and old medication from the eyes with moistened gauze or cotton.

D. Place the child in a sitting or standing position with her head tilted back.

E. Be careful not to touch the dropper to the eye or eyelashes.

F. While the child is looking toward the ceiling, use the index finger and thumb to gently pinch and pull down the lower eyelid to create a "pouch." Drop the prescribed number of drops of the medicine into the pouch and not directly onto the eye.

G. Have the child close her eyes for 1 to 2 minutes.

H. If other eye drops also are prescribed, wait at least 5 minutes before giving the second medicine.

Ointment

A. Wash your hands before giving the medicine.

B. Warm the medicine to **room temperature**.

C. Clean all secretions and old medication from the eyes with moistened gauze or cotton.

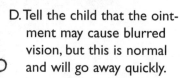

D. Tell the child that the ointment may cause blurred vision, but this is normal and will go away quickly.

E. Place the child on his back with his head tilted back.

F. Be sure not to touch the tip of the tube to the eye or eyelashes.

G. While the child is looking up, gently pull down the lower eyelid. Along the lower eyelid, squeeze out a line of ointment from the inner eye to the outer eye. When reaching the outer eye, rotating the tube will help detach the ointment from the line in the eyelid.

H. Have the child close his eyes for 1 to 2 minutes.

I. Gently wipe any excessive medicine from the eye while it is closed.

J. Before replacing the cap onto the tube, squeeze a small amount of ointment from the tube and discard it. This will help prevent contamination of the medicine.

SKIN MEDICINE

A. Wash your hands.

B. Wash the affected area of skin, unless otherwise directed by a physician, and pat dry with a clean towel.

C. Shake the liquid and aerosolized medicine.

D. Apply the medicine as directed by the physician. If no directions have been provided follow these general guidelines.

   Creams, ointments, gels, solutions, and lotions: usually only a thin layer of the medicine needs to be rubbed onto the skin.

   Aerosol: hold the canister at least 6 inches away from the skin and spray the affected area for several seconds.

E. Be careful not to get any medicine into the child's eyes, ears, or mouth.

F. Wash your hands after the medicine has been applied.

INHALED

Oral Inhaler

A. Remove the cap from the inhaler.

B. Hold the inhaler upright and shake it.

C. Tell the child to breathe out completely (blow out all the air).

D. Administer the medicine by one of the following methods.

E. Clean by soaking in soapy water once a week; rinse and air dry.

1. Inhaler alone

    a. Position inhaler two or three fingers away from the mouth.

    b. While the child slowly breathes in, press on the top of the inhaler to release the medicine.

    c. Tell the child to continue to breathe in until she cannot breathe in any more.

    d. Have the child hold her breath for 10 seconds or as long as she can hold it.

    e. Have the child breathe out slowly.

2.   Inhaler with a spacer

a. Place the inhaler into the spacer, and place the spacer into the child's mouth as shown on the facing page.

b. Press on the top of the inhaler to release the medicine into the spacer.

c. Tell the child to slowly breathe in and out several times, taking deep breaths and holding her breath for several seconds. If the spacer squeaks or whistles while the child is breathing, then she is breathing in or out too fast—tell her to breathe more slowly.

INHALER WITH A SPACER

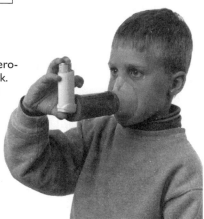

A child using an Aerochamber with face mask. The mask should fit tightly over both the child's mouth and nose. The metallic medicine chamber is kept in its plastic holder and placed at the end of the spacer as shown.

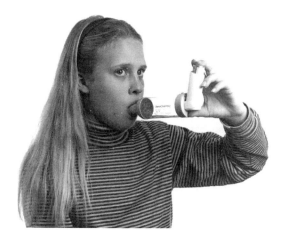

A child using an Aerochamber with mouth piece. The metallic medicine chamber is kept in its plastic holder and placed at the end of the spacer as shown

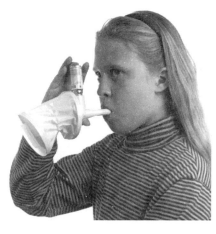

A child using an Inspirease. The metallic medicine chamber is removed from its plastic chamber and placed at the top of the mouth piece as shown.

3. Placing inhaler in mouth

This is the least effective and least favorable way of giving medicine from an inhaler. It must be done only for children who do not have spacers and are not able to accurately squirt the medicine into their mouths from a distance.

a. Directions are the same as those for using an inhaler without a spacer (see item 1, Inhaler alone), except that here the inhaler is placed between the lips (follow steps b, c, d, and e).

E. If more than 1 puff is needed, wait at least 1 minute after the first puff before repeating steps a to d.

F. If multiple medicines from different inhalers are required, it is best to use an inhaled bronchodilator, like albuterol or metaproterenol, before any other.

Capsule Inhaler

A. Place the capsule properly into the inhaler.
Rotahaler: twist the back of the inhaler all the way to the right. Place the small end of the capsule into the opening on the back of the inhaler.
Spinhaler: pull up on the back of the inhaler and remove it. Firmly place the colored end of the capsule into the holder and replace the back of the inhaler.

B. Release the medicine from the capsule.
Rotahaler: twist the back of the inhaler all the way to the left.
Spinhaler: slide the grey sleeve all the way down and then back up.

C. Tell the child to breathe out completely.

D. Tilt her head back slightly and place her lips around the top of the inhaler.

E. Tell the child to inhale quickly and hold her breath for 10 seconds, or for as long as she can.

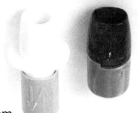

Left: Spinhaler which is used with cromolyn inhaled capsules (Intal).
Right: Rotahaler which is used with albuterol inhaled capsules (Ventolin Rotacaps).

F. Have the child remove the inhaler from her mouth and exhale.

G. Repeat steps C to F until no medicine remains in the inhaler.

H. Clean capsule inhaler by rinsing with water after each use and air drying.

Nebulizer

A. Add the prescribed volume of medicine and diluting liquid into the reservoir (usually a clear plastic cup located at the end of the mouthpiece).

B. Turn the nebulizer on.

C. Be sure a mist is coming out of the mouthpiece before placing it in the child's mouth.

D. Place the end of the mouthpiece into the child's mouth and have the child breathe normally.

E. Unless otherwise directed, the child is finished when there is no more liquid in the reservoir.

F. Clean nebulizer after each use by rinsing the mouthpiece and reservoir with water. Once a week the mouthpiece and reservoir should be soaked in soapy water. Rinse and air dry after cleaning.

NASAL

Drops

A. Have the child gently blow his nose if he is able; an infant suction bulb can be used for babies.

B. Wash your hands before giving the medicine.

C. Position the child according to the following guidelines:

 1. Place an infant lying down in your arms with his head tilted back.

 2. If a child is too large to hold as described above, but is not able to sit upright for the entire procedure, have him lie on his back with a small pillow or other soft item between his shoulders. Then gently tilt his head back.

Nose drops being given to an infant. The infant is lying flat with her head tilted back.

 3. Older children should sit in an upright position with their heads tilted back.

D. Warn the child that he may taste the medicine drops.

E. Warm the medicine to **room temperature** if it is cold.

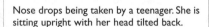

Nose drops being taken by a teenager. She is sitting upright with her head tilted back.

F. Push up gently on the tip of the child's nose.

G. Draw up enough medicine into the dropper so the correct number of drops can be given.

H. Without touching the dropper to the nose, insert the dropper slightly (about one-third of an inch) into the nostril.

I. Instruct the child to breathe through his mouth while the medicine is being placed into his nose.

J. Aim the dropper toward the back of the nostril and squeeze out the prescribed number of drops.

K. Repeat steps F to J if the other nostril needs medicine.

L. After the correct number of drops has been given, tell the child to keep his head tilted back for 5 minutes. Allow him to spit out any medicine that runs down his throat.

M. If the child coughs, place him upright if he is not so. Keep him upright and watch for any problems with his breathing or for excessive coughing. If this occurs, call his physician or the Poison Control Center immediately.

Spray

A. Have the child gently blow his nose if he is able; an infant suction bulb can be used for babies.

B. Have the child sit upright with his head tilted back (as shown).

C. While plugging one nostril, place the tip of the sprayer slightly (about one-half of an inch) into the other nostril.

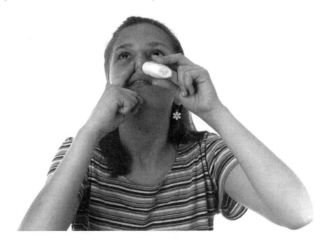

D. While pointing the sprayer straight back and toward the inner corner of the eye, have the child hold his breath.

E. While the child holds his breath, squeeze the sprayer quickly and firmly.

F. The child should continue to hold his breath for several more seconds.

G. Remove the sprayer from the child's nose and allow him to exhale through his mouth.

H. Repeat steps C to G if more sprays are prescribed, or if the other nostril needs medicine.

I. Instruct the child to keep his head tilted back for at least 2 minutes and avoid blowing his nose during this time.

J. Rinse the tip of the sprayer with warm tap water before replacing cap.

Aerosol

A. Have the child gently blow his nose if he is able; an infant suction bulb can be used for babies.

B. Shake the aerosol well and remove the protective cap.

C. Place the tip of the aerosol inside the child's nostril (as shown).

D. While the child holds his breath, firmly press down on the top of the aerosol and then release.

E. The child should continue to hold his breath for at least 3 more seconds.

F. Remove the aerosol from the child's nose and have him exhale through his mouth.

G. If more sprays are prescribed, or if the other nostril needs medication, repeat steps B to F.

H. Instruct the child not to blow his nose for at least 2 minutes after the last spray.

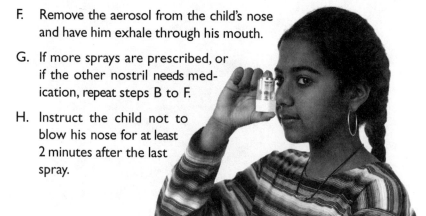

INSULIN INJECTION

A. Make sure the following items are ready to be used:

1. Sterile insulin syringe and needle
2. Vial(s) of insulin
3. Alcohol wipes or rubbing alcohol and gauze or cotton balls

B. Check the label on the insulin vial to be sure the correct type of insulin will be injected. (If the wrong type of insulin is given it increases the risk for too high or too low blood sugar.) Once the correct type of insulin has been confirmed, roll the insulin vial between your hands to mix the medicine. Do not shake the vial.

C. Clean the following areas with an alcohol wipe, gauze, or a cotton ball soaked in rubbing alcohol (do not use the same one to clean both areas):

1. Top of the insulin vial
2. The skin at the site where the injection will be given

D. Remove the protective cap from the needle of the syringe. Pull back on the plunger until the top of the black rubber stopper is at the same number that it will be at after the insulin is drawn into the syringe. This is done so that the same amount of air will be put into the vial that will match the amount of insulin taken out.

E. Place the insulin vial on a hard surface (such as a countertop or table) and insert the needle through the rubber stopper of the vial.

F. Grab both the vial and syringe in one hand and turn them over. (Do not touch the needle.) Push on the plunger with the other hand until all the air is out, then pull it back to the prescribed dose of insulin to be injected (the top of the black rubber stopper should be in the same place as it was in step D).

G. Turn the vial and syringe back over and place the vial back on the hard surface. Pull the syringe out of the vial and turn it over (the needle should be pointing up). Draw any insulin that is in the needle into the syringe by pulling back slightly on the plunger.

H. Examine the insulin inside the syringe. If there are any air bubbles, gently tap the syringe with your finger to move the air bubbles up to the needle. Once all the air bubbles are in the needle, carefully push up on the plunger until liquid just starts to come out of the tip of the needle. This removes all the air bubbles from the syringe and needle.

I. Reexamine the syringe. If any air bubbles remain, pull back on the plunger to put air into the needle and then repeat step H.

J. Pinch the skin at the injection site and hold it. Quickly insert the needle into the skin at a 90-degree angle.

K. Push down on the plunger to inject the insulin. Withdraw the syringe and dispose of it only in proper containers.

RECTAL

Suppository

A. Wash your hands.

B. Have the child lie on his left side; the left leg should be straight and the right leg should be bent up toward his chest.

C. If the suppository is soft, place it under cold running water before unwrapping until it becomes firm. Put on a glove and remove the suppository from its wrapper.

D. With one hand, gently separate the child's buttock cheeks so you can see the rectum.

E. With the other hand, quickly dip the suppository into some cool water or place a small amount of Vaseline or KY Jelly on the tip. Gently insert the smooth, rounded end of the suppository into the rectum.

F. With one finger (use your pinky finger for children younger than 3 years and your index finger for children older than 3 years and adults), push the suppository into the rectum (maximum distance of three inches) until there is no resistance.

G. Remove your finger and check to make sure the suppository is still in the rectum. If it has been inserted far enough the suppository should remain in place. If the suppository comes out, reinsert it into the rectum a little farther than before.

H. If the suppository remains in the rectum, hold the child's buttock cheeks together until the immediate urge to go to the bathroom has passed.

I. Have the child remain in the same position for about 20 minutes. If this becomes a problem, the child should at least sit or lie down for this amount of time, without going to the bathroom.

Ointment

A. Wash your hands and put on gloves.

B. Have the child lie on his left side with the top leg bent up toward his chest.

C. Place the applicator that comes with the ointment onto the end of the tube. Put a small amount of ointment or Vaseline onto the tip of the applicator.

D. With one hand, gently separate the child's buttock cheeks so you can see the rectum.

E. With the other hand, gently insert the applicator into the rectum. Once the applicator is inside, squeeze the tube to insert the prescribed amount of medicine.

F. Remove the applicator from the rectum and the ointment tube and clean it with soap and warm water.

G. Have the child remain in the same position for about 20 minutes. If this becomes a problem, the child should at least sit or lie down for this amount of time, without going to the bathroom.

CALCULATION OF MEDICATION DOSES

In the health profession, the metric system is widely used. Milligrams, grams, or kilograms are used rather than ounces and pounds. Instead of cups or teaspoons for liquid volume, milliliters or liters are used. This section provides a brief introduction to the metric system and dosing of medication in children.

Only a few metric symbols will be needed to help you understand the dosing of medicine. These are summarized in Table 1.

Medicine doses (how much is to be taken) for children usually are calculated based on the child's weight. So, two children who are the same age but different weights may be given different doses of the same medicine.

Can two children of different weights receive the same dose of a medicine? Yes, for several reasons. First, there may not be an appropriate dosage form of the medicine available to provide the correct dose. For example, if a medicine comes as a 250-mg tablet and the dose by weight is 175 mg, the child probably will be given a dose of 250 mg.

Second, medicines have a dosage range, that is, a range in which a particular dose is appropriate. For example, a medicine may have a dosage range of 10–20 milligrams per kilogram of the child's weight (mg/kg). If a 10-kg child and a 20-kg child are each given 200 mg, both doses fall between 10 and 20 mg/kg.

Finally, some medicine doses are based on the "normal" weight of a child at a certain age. That is why some nonprescription medicines state, for example, that children 3–6 years of age receive one dose and children 7–12 years of age receive another. Even though actual weights of children may vary in these age groups, it has been found that an appropriate dose could be given to these groups based on the "normal" weight of children at these ages.

TABLE 1. COMMONLY USED UNITS FOR WEIGHT AND VOLUME

1 pound (lb)	=	2.2	kilograms (kg)
1 kilogram (kg)	=	1000	grams (g)
1 gram (g)	=	1000	milligrams (mg)
1 milligram (mg)	=	1000	micrograms (mcg)
1 teaspoon (tsp)	=	5	milliliters (mL)
1 tablespoon (tbsp)	=	15	milliliters (mL)
1 milliliter (mL)	=	1	cubic centimeter (cc)

Calculation of a dose

Let's take a close look at how you can determine if the child is receiving an appropriate dose of medicine based on the child's weight.

EXAMPLE:

A 44-lb child is given 200 mg of Medicine Z three times a day. The normal dosing range for Medicine Z is 20–40 mg/kg/day divided into equal doses given 3 times a day. How do you calculate the appropriate dose for this child?

The easiest way is by starting with the child's weight and the prescribed dose of the medicine.

1) Convert the child's weight from pounds to kilograms.

$$44 \text{ lb} \div 2.2 = 20 \text{ kg}$$

2) Add all the doses the child gets in one day to determine the total daily dose.

$$200 \text{ mg} \times 3 \text{ times a day} = 600 \text{ mg/day}$$

3) Divide the total daily dose by the child's weight in kilograms.

$$600 \text{ mg/day} \div 20 \text{ kg} = 30 \text{ mg/kg/day}$$

4) Compare the dose calculated in Step 3 to the normal dosing range.

$$\text{Step 3} = 30 \text{ mg/kg/day}$$
$$\text{Normal dosing range} = 20\text{–}40 \text{ mg/kg/day}$$

The dose determined in Step 3 is part of the normal dosage range; therefore, the dose given to the child is appropriate based on weight.

Another method of determining that the child is getting an appropriate dose is by starting with the child's weight and the dosage range of the medicine.

1) Convert the child's weight from pounds to kilograms.

$$44 \text{ lb} \div 2.2 = 20 \text{ kg}$$

2) Calculate the normal high and low daily doses.

Low: 20 mg/kg/day × 20 kg = 400 mg/day

High: 40 mg/kg/day × 20 kg = 800 mg/day

3) Divide the high and low daily doses by the number of times the child receives the medication.

Low: 400 mg/day ÷ 3 times a day = 133 mg/dose

High: 800 mg/day ÷ 3 times a day = 266 mg/dose

4) Compare the dose that the child receives with the calculated high and low doses to see if it falls within the range.

Child's dose: 200 mg 3 times a day

Low dose: 133 mg 3 times a day

High dose: 266 mg 3 times a day

The dose the child receives falls between the calculated high and low doses; therefore, the dose is appropriate based on the child's weight.

Not all medicine doses are based on weight; some are determined by calculating the body surface area (BSA) as measured in square meters (m²). This is accomplished by using the following equation:

$$\text{BSA (m}^2) = \sqrt{\frac{\text{Height (inches)} \times \text{Weight (lb)}}{3131}}$$

Once the body surface area has been calculated, the appropriate dose or dosage range can be calculated by the same methods described above. The only difference in the calculation is that the child's body surface area is used in place of weight.

An example of calculating body surface area and a dose is provided below:

A 50-lb child who is 3'5" tall is to receive 100 mg/m²/day of Medicine Z divided into equal doses given 3 times a day. How much medicine will this child receive with each dose?

1) Calculate body surface area of the child.

Weight: 50 lb

Height: (Must change 3'5" into inches
to fit into the equation.) 3'5" = 41 inches

When a height of 41 inches and weight of 50 lb is placed into the equation, a body surface area of 0.81 m² is calculated.

$$0.81 \ (m^2) \ = \ \sqrt{\dfrac{41 \text{ inches} \times 50 \text{ lb}}{3131}}$$

2) Calculate the total daily dose of the medicine.

100 mg/m²/day × 0.81 m² = 81 mg/day

3) Calculate the individual doses.

81 mg/day ÷ 3 doses/day = 27 mg/dose

READING A MEDICATION PROFILE

Each medicine covered in this book is presented alphabetically in a standard format. We have tried to make it as easy to read and understand as possible. Below is an example of the format used and an explanation of the information in each section. See the example on pages 26 and 27.

① This is the generic name of the medicine. The generic name usually represents the active drug, or combination of drugs, that the medicine contains. There is only one generic name for each medicine.

② Unlike the generic name, a medicine may have many brand names. A brand name is simply the name the company has decided to call the medicine. Brand name products sometimes contain several different drugs. If a brand name product cannot be found in this book, check the listing of active ingredients on the product label.

③ This section states the common uses for which the medicines are prescribed and how they work.

④ This section provides the usual dose of the medicine and the number of times a day it is usually given. Both child and adult doses are provided, since many older children and adolescents may be given the adult dose.

⑤ Listed in this section are oral medications that may interact with the medicine you are giving to cause potentially serious or life-threatening problems. If a potential medication interaction is identified, the child's physician should be notified immediately so that appropriate actions can be taken. If you have any questions about these interactions, a pharmacist also should be able to answer your questions.

This is not a complete list of medication interactions. Always check with the child's physician or a pharmacist for a more extensive list of possible medication interactions.

⑥ The adverse side effects of the medicine are discussed in this section and are divided into two categories: minor and severe.

Minor adverse side effects are the less serious ones that may be observed in some people taking the medicine. Attention to minor adverse side effects is necessary since these can possibly be harmful. An example of this is sedation. This side effect is common with many medicines, but usually is considered to be minor. However, if the child is playing on the swing set while experiencing sedation from the medicine, she may be seriously injured by falling off the swing. Even though the side effect may be minor, the child's physician should always be notified if one occurs.

Severe adverse side effects are usually rare, but can be life-threatening or be signs of a more serious problem. An example of this is unusual bruising or bleeding. This side effect may seem mild, but it may indicate that a condition called thrombocytopenia (low platelet count) has developed. Platelets are used by the body to stop bleeding. If the platelet count goes too low, the child could possibly bleed to death from a minor injury. Even though these side effects do not occur very often, if adverse side effects designated as "severe" occur, the child's physician should be notified as soon as possible.

⑦ This section discusses the proper storage and administration of the medicine. The answers to a variety of questions, such as whether the medicine should be refrigerated, crushed, mixed with fruit juice, or taken with food, can be found here.

⑧ The special instruction section contains directions that should be followed while the child is receiving the medicine, what may be done to prevent some common adverse side effects, and so on.

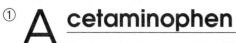

① # Acetaminophen (SAMPLE PROFILE)

(See the explanation on pages 24 and 25).

(See the explanation on pages 24 and 25).

② ## Brand Names

Acephen
(rectal
suppository)

Acetaminophen
Uniserts
(rectal
suppository)

Anacin–3
(tablet)

Children's
Anacin–3
(chewable
tablet, liquid)

Children's
Feverall
(rectal
suppository)

Children's
Panadol
(chewable
tablet, liquid)

Children's
Tylenol
(chewable
tablet, liquid)

(continued next page)

③ ## Common Uses

Acetaminophen is a medicine used to relieve fever and mild-to-moderate pain. It blocks the production of chemicals in the brain responsible for pain and also affects the temperature-regulating center of the brain. Acetaminophen does not relieve inflammation. Therefore, it may not relieve all the pain due to arthritis or other joint or tissue inflammatory disease.

④ ## Usual Dose

TABLET, CHEWABLE TABLET, CAPSULE, AND LIQUID

Children younger than 12 years: 10–15 mg/kg/dose given every 4–6 hours as needed for pain or fever. Maximum dose 5 g/day.

Children older than 12 years and Adults: 325–650 mg/dose given every 4–6 hours or 1000 mg/dose every 6–8 hours as needed for pain or fever. Maximum dose 4 g/day.

RECTAL SUPPOSITORY See the Medication Administration section for instructions on the proper use of a rectal suppository (page 19).

Children 3–6 years old: 120 mg/dose given every 4–6 hours as needed for fever. Maximum dose 720 mg/day.

Children 6–12 years old: 325 mg/dose given every 4–6 hours as needed for fever. Maximum dose 2600 mg/day.

Adults: 650 mg/dose given every 4–6 hours as needed for fever. Maximum of 6 doses a day.

⑤ ## Medication Interactions

Acetaminophen may decrease the effectiveness of:

rimantadine

Medications that increase the risk for the development of liver toxicity when combined with acetaminophen are:

alcohol

phenytoin

sulfinpyrazone

⑥ Adverse Side Effects

Minor: Dizziness, trembling.

Severe: Fatigue, rash, hives, sore throat, fever, blood in the urine, unusual bruising or bleeding, yellow skin or eyes.

⑦ Storage and Administration

The oral medicine should be stored in a cool, dry place away from light. Prolonged exposure to heat, moisture, or light can damage the medicine.

The liquid may be stored at room temperature and does not need to be refrigerated.

Refrigeration of the rectal suppositories is recommended.

If upset stomach occurs, the medicine can be given with food.

The chewable tablet should be chewed thoroughly before swallowing.

If the child is unable to swallow pills, the nonchewable tablets can be crushed or the capsules opened and mixed with a small amount of water or soft food (such as applesauce, pudding, jam, or jelly). This mixture should be swallowed and not chewed. The entire mixture must be swallowed to ensure that the child received the full dose.

Even though liquid acetaminophen does not taste bad, some children may not want to take it. If this occurs, the liquid medicine can be disguised by mixing the dose with water or juice. The entire mixture must be swallowed to ensure that the child received the full dose.

⑧ Special Instructions

The child's physician should be notified if the pain or fever is not relieved by the medicine.

Brand Names ②

(continued)

Junior Strength Feverall (rectal suppository)

Neopap (rectal suppository)

Panadol (tablet)

St. Joseph Aspirin-Free (chewable tablet, liquid)

Suppap-120 (rectal suppository)

Suppap-325 (rectal suppository)

Suppap-650 (rectal suppository)

Tempra (chewable tablet, liquid)

Tylenol (capsule, tablet, liquid)

MEDICATIONS AND BREAST FEEDING

Breast feeding is a natural, safe, effective, and preferred way of providing the nutrition required for a newborn baby to grow and stay healthy. Unfortunately, it also may be a way for the baby to be exposed to medicines that the mother is taking. It is best for the mother to not take any medicines while breast feeding, but this is not possible when one has an acute or chronic disease requiring medications.

This section is a guide to whether the medicine that the mother is taking may or may not harm the baby. Even if the medicine is listed as safe for use during breast feeding, adverse side effects still may occur in the infant. Much of the information to determine whether a medicine is safe comes from reports of its use in a few infants who are breast fed or an estimation of how much of the medication an infant would receive if breast milk was ingested. It is always important to watch for adverse side effects of the medicines in the infant, which are listed in this book. (If the medicine is not listed in the tables presented here, check the index to see if the medicine is listed under another name.) If the medicine is not listed in this book, ask the prescribing physician or pharmacist about the possible adverse side effects that you should watch for in the baby. Always report any changes in the child's looks or behavior to her physician to determine whether the changes may be related to the medicine in the breast milk.

Not all medicines that may be taken by a mother are listed here. Just because a medicine is not listed does not mean that it is safe to take. Contact your physician or pharmacist to check if breast feeding is allowed while you take this medication.

MEDICATIONS AND DRUGS OF ABUSE THAT SHOULD <u>NEVER</u> BE USED WHEN AN INFANT IS BREAST FEEDING

Amphetamine	Lithium
Bromocriptine	Marijuana
Cocaine	Methotrexate
Cyclosporine	Nicotine (smoking)
Ergotamine	Phencyclidine (PCP)
Heroin	

MEDICATIONS THAT MAY CAUSE PROBLEMS IN NURSING INFANTS

IF THESE MEDICATIONS HAVE BEEN PRESCRIBED THEY SHOULD BE USED WITH CAUTION AND UNDER THE SUPERVISION OF A PHYSICIAN

Acebutolol	Labetalol
Alcohol	Lead
Aloin	Lincomycin
Alprazolam	Lindane
Amiodarone	Lomefloxacin
Amitriptyline	Lorazepam
Amoxapine	Mesoridazine
Aspirin	Methadone[a]
Atenolol	Methylergonovine
Carbamazepine	Metoclopramide
Chloral hydrate	Metoprolol
Chloramphenicol	Metronidazole[b]
Chlorpromazine	Minocycline
Chlorprothixene	Morphine
Cimetidine	Nadolol
Ciprofloxacin	Norfloxacin
Clemastine fumarate	Nortriptyline
Codeine	Ofloxacin
Cyproheptadine	Pentobarbital
Demeclocycline	Perphenazine
Desipramine	Phenobarbital
Diazepam	Prazepam
Dothiepin	Primidone
Doxepin	Quazepam
Doxycycline	Quinidine
Enoxacin	Sotalol
Ergonovine	Sulfasalazine
Fluoxetine	Temazepam
Ginseng	Tetracycline
Haloperidol	Theophylline
Imipramine	Timolol
Iodine	Trazodone

[a]If the mother receives more than 20 mg/day of methadone.
[b]If the mother receives a single, 2-g dose of metronidazole, the breast milk should be pumped and discarded for 24 hours after the dose is taken. Breast feeding may be restarted after this.

Medications That Are Generally Considered to be Safe When Used During Breast Feeding

Acetaminophen	Disopyramide
Acetazolamide	Domperidone
Acitretin	Enalapril
Acyclovir	Epinephrine
Allopurinol	Erythromycin
Amoxicillin	Estradiol
Ampicillin	Ethambutol
Atropine	Ethosuximide
Baclofen	Famotidine
Bendroflu-	Flecainide
methiazide	Fluoride
Bretylium	Flurbiprofen
Butabarbital	Folic acid
Caffeine	Furosemide
Captopril	Hydralazine
Carbimazole	Hydrochlorothiazide
Cefadroxil	Hydroxychloroquine sulfate
Cefprozil	Ibuprofen
Cephalexin	Indomethacin
Cephradine	Insulin
Chloroquine	Isoniazid
Chlorothiazide	Kanamycin
Chlorthalidone	Ketorolac
Cisapride	Levonorgestrel
Clindamycin	Loperamide
Clomipramine	Magnesium hydroxide
Clonazepam	Medroxyprogesterone
Clonidine	Mefenamic acid
Colchicine	Mestranol
Cyanocobalamin	Methadone[a]
Cycloserine	Methimazole
Danthron	Methocarbamol
Dapsone	Methyldopa
Desmopressin	Methyprylon
Dicumarol	Mexiletine
Digoxin	Mineral oil
Diltiazem	Minoxidil

[a]If the mother receives less than 20 mg/day of methadone.

MEDICATIONS THAT ARE GENERALLY CONSIDERED TO BE SAFE WHEN USED DURING BREAST FEEDING

Nalidixic acid
Naproxen
Nifedipine
Nitrofurantoin
Nizatidine
Norethynodrel
Noscapine
Oxazepam
Oxycodone
Penicillin G potassium
Penicillin V potassium
Pentoxifylline
Phenolphthalein
Phenylbutazone
Phenytoin
Phytonadione
Piroxicam
Prednisolone[b]
Prednisone[b]
Procainamide
Progesterone
Propoxyphene
Propranolol
Propylthiouracil
Pseudoephedrine
Pyrazinamide
Pyridostigmine

Pyridoxine
Pyrimethamine
Quinine sulfate
Ranitidine
Riboflavin
Rifampin
Scopolamine
Secobarbital
 sodium
Senna
Spironolactone
Sulfanilamide[c]
Sulfathiazole[c]
Sulfisoxazole[c]
Terbutaline
Thiamine
Tocainide
Tolbutamide
Tolmetin
Trimethoprim
Triprolidine
Valproic acid
Verapamil
Vitamin D
Warfarin sodium
Zolpidem tartrate

[b]If the mother receives more than 20 mg/day, she should wait 3–4 hours after each dose before breast feeding.
[c]These medications should be used with caution in infants that are ill, stressed, premature, or have hyperbilirubinemia (high concentration of bilirubin in the blood) or glucose-6-phosphate dehydrogenase deficiency.

(Continued from previous page)

BRAND NAME DRUG REFERENCES

A

Acephen*
see Acetaminophen, 48

Acetaminophen Uniserts*
see Acetaminophen, 48

Achromycin*
see Tetracycline hydrochloride, 311

Achromycin V*
see Tetracycline hydrochloride, 311

Actidil*
see Triprolidine, 31

Adalat*
see Nifedipine, 246

Adapin*
see Doxepin, 29

Advil*
see Ibuprofen, 207

AeroBid
see Flunisolide, 187

AeroBid M
see Flunisolide, 187

Aerolate*
see Theophylline, 315

Aerolate JR*
see Theophylline, 315

Aerolate SR*
see Theophylline, 315

Aeroseb-Dex
see Dexamethasone, 137

Aeroseb-HC
see Hydrocortisone, 204

AK-Dex
see Dexamethasone, 137

Ala-Cort
see Hydrocortisone, 204

Ala-Scalp
see Hydrocortisone, 204

Aldactone*
see Spironolactone, 299

Aldomet*
see Methyldopa, 30

Aleve*
see Naproxen, 244

Aller-Chlor
see Chlorpheniramine maleate, 105

AllerMax Caplets
see Diphenhydramine hydrochloride, 154

Allermed*
see Pseudoephedrine hydrochloride, 287

Alupent
see Metaproterenol sulfate, 230

Ambien*
see Zolpidem tartrate, 31

Amen*
see Medroxyprogesterone, 30

Amodopa*
see Methyldopa, 30

Amoxil*
see Amoxicillin, 62

Anacin-3*
see Acetaminophen, 48

Anafranil*
see Clomipramine, 30

Anaprox*
see Naproxen, 244

Anaprox DS*
see Naproxen, 244

Ansaid*
see Flurbiprofen, 30

Anti-Tuss
see Guaifenesin, 195

Anusol-HC 2.5%
see Hydrocortisone, 204

Apresoline*
see Hydralazine hydrochloride, 200

Aquachloral Supprettes*
see Chloral hydrate, 29

Aquaphyllin*
see Theophylline, 315

Aralen*
see Chloroquine, 30

Aristocort
see Triamcinolone, 326

Aristocort A
see Triamcinolone, 326

Asendin*
see Amoxapine, 29

AsthmaHaler Mist
see Epinephrine, 163

AsthmaNefrin
see Epinephrine, 163

Ativan*
see Lorazepam, 29

Atolone
see Triamcinolone, 326

Augmentin
see Amoxicillin and Clavulanic acid, **64**

*There is information on these medications (listed by generic name) in the section on Medications and Breast Feeding (page 28).

AVC*
see Sulfanilamide, 31

Aventyl*
see Nortriptyline, 29

Axid Pulvules*
see Nizatidine, 31

Azmacort
see Triamcinolone, 326

Azolid*
see Phenylbutazone, 31

AZT
see Zidovudine, 341

Azulfidine*
see Sulfasalazine, 29

Azulfidine EN-tabs*
see Sulfasalazine, 29

B

Bactine Hydrocortisone
see Hydrocortisone, 204

Bactocill
see Oxacillin sodium, 252

Bactrim
see Trimethoprim with Sulfamethoxazole, 332

Bactrim DS
see Trimethoprim with Sulfamethoxazole, 332

Banophen
see Diphenhydramine hydrochloride, 154

Banophen Caplets
see Diphenhydramine hydrochloride, 154

Bayer Children's Aspirin*
see Aspirin, 29

Beclovent
see Beclomethasone, 76

Beconase
see Beclomethasone, 76

Beconase AQ
see Beclomethasone, 76

Beepen-VK*
see Penicillin V potassium, 262

Belix
see Diphenhydramine hydrochloride, 154

Benadryl
see Diphenhydramine hydrochloride, 154

Benadryl 25
see Diphenhydramine hydrochloride, 154

Benylin Cough
see Diphenhydramine hydrochloride, 154

Benylin DM
see Dextromethorphan, 144

Betapace*
see Sotalol, 29

Betapen VK*
see Penicillin V potassium, 262

Biaxin
see Clarithromycin, 116

Biomox*
see Amoxicillin, 62

Blocadren*
see Timolol, 29

Brethaire*
see Terbutaline sulfate, 307

Brethine*
see Terbutaline sulfate, 307

Bretylol*
see Bretylium, 30

Bricanyl*
see Terbutaline sulfate, 307

Bromphen
see Brompheniramine maleate, 82

Bronitin Mist
see Epinephrine, 163

Bronkaid Mist
see Epinephrine, 163

Bronkodyl*
see Theophylline, 315

Bufferin*
see Aspirin, 29

Buffex*
see Aspirin, 29

Butazolidin*
see Phenylbutazone, 31

Butisol*
see Butabarbital, 30

Caffedrine*
see Caffeine, 30

Calan*
see Verapamil, 31

Calan SR*
see Verapamil, 31

Capital with Codeine
see Acetaminophen with Codeine, 50

Capoten*
see Captopril, 84

Carafate
see Sucralfate, 84

Cardioquin*
see Quinidine, 29

Cardizem*
see Diltiazem, 30

Cardizem CD*
see Diltiazem, 30

Cardizem SR*
see Diltiazem, 30

Catapres*
see *Clonidine, 30*

Ceclor
see *Cefaclor, 89*

Ceftin
see *Cefuroxime axetil, 99*

Cefzil*
see *Cefprozil, 97*

Cenafed*
see *Pseudoephedrine hydrochloride, 287*

Centrax*
see *Prazepam, 29*

Cetacort
see *Hydrocortisone, 204*

Children's Anacin-3*
see *Acetaminophen, 48*

Children's Feverall*
see *Acetaminophen, 48*

Children's Hold
see *Dextromethorphan, 144*

Children's Panadol*
see *Acetaminophen, 48*

Children's Sudafed*
see *Pseudoephedrine hydrochloride, 287*

Children's Tylenol*
see *Acetaminophen, 48*

Chlo-Amine
see *Chlorpheniramine maleate, 105*

Chlorate
see *Chlorpheniramine maleate, 105*

Chloromycetin Kapseals*
see *Chloramphenicol, 29*

Chloromycetin Palmitate*
see *Chloramphenicol, 29*

Chlortab-4
see *Chlorpheniramine maleate, 105*

Chlortab-8
see *Chlorpheniramine maleate, 105*

Chlor-Trimeton
see *Chlorpheniramine maleate, 105*

Chlor-Trimeton Repetabs
see *Chlorpheniramine maleate, 105*

Ciloxan*
see *Ciprofloxacin, 114*

Cipro*
see *Ciprofloxacin, 114*

Cleocin*
see *Clindamycin hydrochloride, 118*

Cleocin T*
see *Clindamycin hydrochloride, 118*

Cloxapen
see *Cloxacillin sodium, 124*

Coffee Break Caplets*
see *Caffeine, 30*

Cogentin
see *Benztropine mesylate, 78*

Cordarone*
see *Amiodarone, 29*

Corgard*
see *Nadolol, 29*

CortaGel
see *Hydrocortisone, 204*

Cortaid
see *Hydrocortisone, 204*

Cort-Dome
see *Hydrocortisone, 204*

Cortef
see *Hydrocortisone, 204*

Cortizone•5
see *Hydrocortisone, 204*

Cortizone•10
see *Hydrocortisone, 204*

Cotazym
see *Pancrelipase, 256*

Cotazym-S
see *Pancrelipase, 256*

Cotrim
see *Trimethoprim with Sulfamethoxazole, 332*

Cotrim D.S.
see *Trimethoprim with Sulfamethoxazole, 332*

Cotrim Pediatric
see *Trimethoprim with Sulfamethoxazole, 332*

Co-trimoxazole
see *Trimethoprim with Sulfamethoxazole, 332*

Coumadin*
see *Warfarin sodium, 336*

Curretab*
see *Medroxyprogesterone, 30*

Cycrin*
see *Medroxyprogesterone, 30*

Cylert
see *Pemoline, 258*

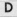

D

Daraprim*
see *Pyrimethamine, 31*

Darvon Pulvules*
see *Propoxyphene, 31*

Dazamide*
see *Acetazolamide, 30*

DDAVP*
see *Desmopressin, 30*

ddC
see *Zalcitabine, 339*

ddI
see *Didanosine, 148*

Decadron
see *Dexamethasone, 137*

Decadron Phosphate Respihaler
see *Dexamethasone, 137*

Decadron Phosphate Turbinaire
see *Dexamethasone, 137*

Decaspray
see *Dexamethasone, 137*

Declomycin*
see *Demeclocycline, 29*

Decofed*
see *Pseudoephedrine hydrochloride, 287*

Delsym
see *Dextromethorphan, 144*

Delta-Cortef*
see *Prednisolone, 273*

Deltasone*
see *Prednisone, 275*

Delta-Tritex
see *Triamcinolone, 326*

Depakene*
see *Valproic acid, 334*

Depakote*
see *Divalproex sodium, 156*

Dermolate
see *Hydrocortisone, 204*

Desyrel*
see *Trazodone hydrochloride, 324*

Dexameth
see *Dexamethasone, 137*

Dexamethasone Intensol
see *Dexamethasone, 137*

Dexedrine
see *Dextroamphetamine, 142*

Dexedrine Spansules
see *Dextroamphetamine, 142*

Dexone
see *Dexamethasone, 142*

Diamine T.D.
see *Brompheniramine maleate, 82*

Diamox*
see *Acetazolamide, 30*

Diamox Sequels*
see *Acetazolamide, 30*

Diflucan
see *Fluconazole, 185*

Dilacor XR*
see *Diltiazem, 30*

Dilantin 30 Pediatric*
see *Phenytoin sodium, 270*

Dilantin 125*
see *Phenytoin sodium, 270*

Dilantin Infatab*
see *Phenytoin sodium, 270*

Dilantin Kapseals*
see *Phenytoin sodium, 270*

Diltiazem Extended Release*
see *Diltiazem, 30*

Dimetane
see *Brompheniramine maleate, 82*

Dimetane Extentabs
see *Brompheniramine maleate, 82*

Diphenylan sodium*
see *Phenytoin sodium, 270*

Ditropan
see *Oxybutynin, 254*

Diurigen*
see *Chlorothizide, 30*

Diuril*
see *Chlorothizide, 30*

Dolene*
see *Propoxyphene, 31*

Dolophine*
see *Methadone, 30*

Doral*
see *Quazepam, 29*

Dorbane*
see *Danthron, 30*

Dorcol Children's Decongestant*
see *Pseudoephedrine hydrochloride, 287*

Dormarex 2
see *Diphenhydramine hydrochloride, 154*

Doryx*
see *Doxycycline, 158*

Doxy Caps*
see *Doxycycline, 158*

Doxychel Hyclate*
see *Doxycycline, 158*

Duricef*
see *Cefadroxil, 91*

Duvoid
see *Bethanechol chloride, 80*

Dycill
see *Dicloxacillin sodium, 146*

Dynapen
see *Dicloxacillin sodium, 146*

E

Ecotrin*
see *Aspirin, 29*

E.E.S. 200*
see *Erythromycin ethylsuccinate, 169*

E.E.S. 400*
see *Erythromycin ethylsuccinate, 169*

E.E.S. Granules*
see *Erythromycin ethylsuccinate, 169*

Elavil*
see *Amitriptyline hydrochloride, 59*

Elimit
see *Permethrin, 264*

Elixophyllin*
see *Theophylline, 315*

Empirin*
see Aspirin, 29

E-Mycin*
see Erythromycin base, 165

Endep*
see Amitriptyline hydrochloride, 59

Enovid*
see Mestranol, 30, and Norethynodrel, 31

Epipen
see Epinephrine, 163

Epipen Jr.
see Epinephrine, 163

Epitol*
see Carbamazepine, 86

Eramycin*
see Erythromycin stearate, 171

Ergostat*
see Ergotamine, 28

Ergotrate*
see Ergonovine, 29

Eryc*
see Erythromycin base, 165

EryPed*
see Erythromycin ethylsuccinate, 169

EryPed 200*
see Erythromycin ethylsuccinate, 169

EryPed 400*
see Erythromycin ethylsuccinate, 169

Ery-Tab*
see Erythromycin base, 165

Erythrocin Stearate*
see Erythromycin stearate, 171

Eryzol
see Erythromycin with Sulfisoxazole, 173

Eskalith*
see Lithium, 28

Eskalith CR*
see Lithium, 28

Esidrix*
see Hydrochlorothiazide, 202

Espotabs*
see Phenolphthalein, 31

Estrace*
see Estradiol, 30

Estraderm*
see Estradiol, 30

Evac-U-Gen*
see Phenolphthalein, 31

Excedrin IB*
see Ibuprofen, 207

Ex-Lax*
see Phenolphthalein, 31

F

Feen-a-mint*
see Phenolphthalein, 31

Felbatol
see Felbamate, 179

Feldene*
see Piroxicam, 31

Feosol
see Ferrous sulfate, 183

Feratab
see Ferrous sulfate, 183

Fergon
see Ferrous gluconate, 181

Fer-In-Sol
see Ferrous sulfate, 183

Ferndex
see Dextroamphetamine, 142

Fero-Gradumet Filmtab
see Ferrous sulfate, 183

Ferospace
see Ferrous sulfate, 183

Ferralet
see Ferrous gluconate, 181

Ferralet Slow Release
see Ferrous gluconate, 181

Ferralyn Lanacaps
see Ferrous sulfate, 183

Ferra-TD
see Ferrous sulfate, 183

Flagyl*
see Metronidazole, 237

Floxin*
see Ofloxacin, 29

Flumadine
see Rimantadine hydrochloride, 297

Fluoritab*
see Fluoride, 30

Flura*
see Fluoride, 30

Flura-Drops*
see Fluoride, 30

Flura-Loz*
see Fluoride, 30

Flutex
see Triamcinolone, 326

Formula Q*
see Quinine sulfate, 31

Furadantin*
see Nitrofurantoin, 248

Furalan*
see Nitrofurantoin, 248

Furanite*
see Nitrofurantoin, 248

Gantanol
see Sulfamethoxazole, 303

Gantrisin*
see Sulfisoxazole, 305

Gastrocrom
see Cromolyn sodium, 128

Genahist
see Diphenhydramine hydrochloride, 154

Genaphed*
see Pseudoephedrine hydrochloride, 287

Genprin*
see Aspirin, 29

Glyate
see Guaifenesin, 195

Guiatuss
see Guaifenesin, 195

G-well*
see Lindane, 226

Haldol*
see Haloperidol, 197

Halofed*
see Pseudoephedrine hydrochloride, 287

Halotussin
see Guaifenesin, 195

1% HC
see Hydrocortisone, 204

Hexadrol
see Dexamethasone, 137

Hismanal
see Astemizole, 70

Hivid
see Zalcitabine, 339

Hold DM
see Dextromethorphan, 144

Humibid L.A.
see Guaifenesin, 195

Humibid Sprinkle
see Guaifenesin, 195

Humulin 70/30*
see Insulin, 215

Humulin L*
see Insulin, 215

Humulin N*
see Insulin, 215

Humulin R*
see Insulin, 215

Hycort
see Hydrocortisone, 204

Hydramine
see Diphenhydramine hydrochloride, 154

HydroDIURIL*
see Hydrochlorothiazide, 202

Hydro-Par*
see Hydrochlorothiazide, 202

HydroTex
see Hydrocortisone, 204

Hygroton*
see Chlorthalidone, 30

Hytone
see Hydrocortisone, 204

Hytuss
see Guaifenesin, 195

Hytuss 2X
see Guaifenesin, 195

I, J, K

Ibuprin*
see Ibuprofen, 207

Ilosone*
see Erythromycin estolate, 167

Ilozyme
see Pancrelipase, 256

Imodium*
see Loperamide, 30

Imodium A-D*
see Loperamide, 30

Imodium A-D Caplets*
see Loperamide, 30

Inderal*
see Propranolol hydrochloride, 283

Inderal LA*
see Propranolol hydrochloride, 283

Indocin*
see Indomethacin, 213

Indocin SR*
see Indomethacin, 213

Indomethacin SR*
see Indomethacin, 213

Intal
see Cromolyn sodium, 128

Iodo-Niacin*
see Iodine, 29

Isoptin*
see Verapamil, 31

Isoptin SR*
see Verapamil, 31

Istizin*
see Danthron, 30

Janimine*
see Imipramine hydrochloride, 210

Junior Strength Feverall*
see Acetaminophen, 48

Kantrex*
see Kanamycin, 30

Kaopectate II Caplets*
see Loperamide, 30

Karidium*
see Fluoride, 30

Keflet*
see Cephalexin, 101

Keflex*
see Cephalexin, 101

Keftab*
see Cephalexin, 101

Kenacort
see Triamcinolone, 326

Kenalog
see Triamcinolone, 326

Kenalog-H
see Triamcinolone, 326

Kenonel
see Triamcinolone, 326

Klonopin*
see Clonazepam, 120

Kondremul Plain*
see Mineral oil, 30

Kwell*
see Lindane, 226

Ku-Zyme
see Pancrelipase, 256

L

Laniazid*
see Isoniazid, 217

Laniazid C.T.*
see Isoniazid, 217

Lanophyllin*
see Theophylline, 315

Lanoxicaps*
see Digoxin, 151

Lanoxin*
see Digoxin, 151

Lasix
see Furosemide, 191

Lax Pills*
see Phenolphthalein, 31

Laxative Pills*
see Phenolphthalein, 31

Ledercillin VK*
see Penicillin V potassium, 262

Legatrin*
see Quinine sulfate, 31

Lente Insulin*
see Insulin, 215

Levothroid
see Levothyroxine sodium, 224

Levoxine
see Levothyroxine sodium, 224

Lincocin*
see Lincomycin, 29

Lioresal*
see Baclofen, 30

Liquid Pred*
see Prednisone, 275

Lithane*
see Lithium, 28

Lithobid*
see Lithium, 28

Lithonate*
see Lithium, 28

Lithotabs*
see Lithium, 28

Loniten*
see Minoxidil, 30

Lopressor*
see Metoprolol, 29

Lorabid
see Loracarbef, 228

Lotrimin
see Clotrimazole, 122

Lotrimin AF
see Clotrimazole, 122

Lugol's Solution*
see Iodine, 29

Luride Lozi-Tabs*
see Fluoride, 30

M

M-KYA*
see Quinine sulfate, 31

Macrodantin*
see Nitrofurantoin, 248

Magnaprin*
see Aspirin, 29

Magnesium hydroxide,* 30

Maxaquin*
see Lomefloxacin, 29

Maxidex
see Dexamethasone, 137

Medihaler-Epi
see Epinephrine, 163

Medilax*
see Phenolphthalein, 31

Medipren*
see Ibuprofen, 207

Mellaril
see Thioridazine hydrochloride, 318

Mellaril S
see Thioridazine hydrochloride, 318

Mephyton*
see Phytonadione, 31

Mestinon*
see Pyridostigmine, 31

Metaprel
see Metaproterenol sulfate, 230

Methadone Intensol*
see Methadone, 30

Methergine*
see Methylergonovine, 29

Meticorten*
see Prednisone, 275

MetroGel*
see Metronidazole, 237

Mexitil*
see Mexiletine, 30

Midol 200*
see Ibuprofen, 207

Milk of Magnesia*
see Magnesium hydroxide, 30

Milkinol*
see Mineral oil, 30

Minocin*
see Minocycline hydrochloride, 240

Mol-Iron
see Ferrous sulfate, 183

Motilium*
see Domperidone, 30

Motrin IB*
see Ibuprofen, 207

MS Contin*
see Morphine, 29

MSIR*
see Morphine, 29

Myambutol*
see Ethambutol, 175

Mycelex
see Clotrimazole, 122

Mycostatin
see Nystatin, 250

Mycostatin Pastilles
see Nystatin, 250

Myidyl*
see Triprolidine, 31

Myotonachol
see Bethanechol chloride, 80

Mysoline*
see Primidone, 277

Mytussin
see Guaifenesin, 195

N, O

Naprosyn*
see Naproxen, 244

Nasacort
see Triamcinolone, 326

Nasalcrom
see Cromolyn sodium, 128

Nasalide
see Flunisolide, 187

Naturetin*
see Bendroflumethiazide, 30

Navane
see Thiothixene, 321

NegGram*
see Naldixic acid, 31

Nembutal*
see Pentobarbital, 29

Neo-mercazole*
see Carbimazole, 30

Neopap*
see Acetaminophen, 48

Nestrex*
see Pyridoxine, 31

Neurontin
see Gabapentin, 193

Nilstat
see Nystatin, 250

Nitrofan*
see Nitrofurantoin, 248

Nix
see Permethrin, 264

Nizoral
see Ketoconazole, 220

Noctec*
see Chloral hydrate, 29

NoDoz*
see Caffeine, 30

Noludar*
see Methyprylon, 30

Normodyne*
see Labetalol, 29

Noroxin*
see Norfloxacin, 29

Norpace*
see Disopyramide, 30

Norpace CR*
see Disopyramide, 30

Norplant*
see Levonorgestrel, 30

Norpramin*
see Desipramine hydrochloride, 134

Nor-Tet*
see Tetracycline hydrochloride, 311

Norwich Aspirin*
see Aspirin, 29

Novafed*
see Pseudoephedrine hydrochloride, 287

Novolin 70/30*
see Insulin, 215

Novolin L*
see Insulin, 215

Novolin N*
see Insulin, 215

Novolin R*
see Insulin, 215

NPH Insulin*
see Insulin, 215

Nuprin*
see Ibuprofen, 207

Nutracort
see Hydrocortisone, 204

Nystex
see Nystatin, 250

Omnipen*
see Ampicillin, 68

Opticrom
see Cromolyn sodium, 128

Orasone*
see Prednisone, 275

Oretic*
see Hydrochlorothiazide, 202

Orinase*
see Tolbutamide, 31

P

Pamelor*
see Nortriptyline, 29

Pamprin-IB*
see Ibuprofen, 207

Panadol*
see Acetaminophen, 48

Panasol-S*
see Prednisone, 275

Pancrease
see Pancrelipase, 256

Pancrease MT4
see Pancrelipase, 256

Pancrease MT10
see Pancrelipase, 256

Pancrease MT16
see Pancrelipase, 256

Panmycin*
see Tetracycline hydrochloride, 311

Panwarfin*
see Warfarin sodium, 336

Parlodel*
see Bromocriptine, 28

Parlodel SnapTabs*
see Bromocriptine, 28

Pathocil
see Dicloxacillin sodium, 146

PCE Dispertab*
see Erythromycin base, 165

PediaCare Infant's Decongestant*
see Pseudoephedrine hydrochloride, 287

Pediaflor*
see Fluoride, 30

Pediapred*
see Prednisolone, 273

PediaProfen*
see Ibuprofen, 207

Pediazole
see Erythromycin with Sulfisoxazole, 173

Penetrex*
see Enoxacin, 29

Penicillin VK*
see Penicillin V potassium, 262

Pentids*
see Penicillin G potassium, 260

Pen-Vee K*
see Penicillin V potassium, 262

Pepcid*
see Famotidine, 30

Pepto Diarrhea Control*
see Loperamide, 30

Periactin*
see Cyproheptadine, 29

Pertofrane*
see Desipramine hydrochloride, 134

Pertussin CS
see Dextromethorphan, 144

Pertussin ES
see Dextromethorphan, 144

Pharmaflur*
see Fluoride, 30

Phenameth
see Promethazine hydrochloride, 281

Phenaphen with Codeine
see Acetaminophen with Codeine, 50

Phencyclidine (PCP),* 28

Phendry
see Diphenhydramine hydrochloride, 154

Phenergan
see Promethazine hydrochloride, 281

Phenetron
see Chlorpheniramine maleate, 105

Phenolax*
see Phenolphthalein, 31

Phillips' Chewable*
see *Magnesium hydroxide, 30*

Phillips' Milk of Magnesia*
see *Magnesium hydroxide, 30*

Pima*
see *Iodine, 29*

Plaquenil sulfate*
see *Hydroxychloroquine sulfate, 30*

Polycillin*
see *Ampicillin, 68*

Polymox*
see *Amoxicillin, 68*

Ponstel*
see *Mefenamic acid, 30*

Potassium iodide*
see *Iodine, 29*

Prednicen-M*
see *Prednisone, 275*

Prednisone Intensol*
see *Prednisone, 275*

Prelone*
see *Prednisolone, 273*

Primatene Mist
see *Epinephrine, 163*

Principen*
see *Ampicillin, 68*

Procan SR*
see *Procainamide hydrochloride, 279*

Procardia*
see *Nifedipine, 246*

Procardia XL*
see *Nifedipine, 246*

Proctocort
see *Hydrocortisone, 204*

Progestasert*
see *Progesterone, 31*

Proloprim*
see *Trimethoprim, 31*

Pronestyl*
see *Procainamide hydrochloride, 279*

Pronestyl-SR*
see *Procainamide hydrochloride, 279*

Propagest
see *Phenylpropanolamine hydrochloride, 268*

Propulsid*
see *Cisapride, 30*

Propranolol Hydrochloride Intensol* see *Propranolol hydrochloride, 283*

Prostaphlin
see *Oxacillin sodium, 252*

Prothiaden*
see *Dothiepin, 29*

Protilase
see *Pancrelipase, 256*

Protostat*
see *Metronidazole, 237*

Proventil
see *Albuterol, 54*

Proventil Repetabs
see *Albuterol, 54*

Provera*
see *Medroxyprogesterone, 30*

Prozac*
see *Fluoxetine hydrochloride, 189*

Pseudo*
see *Pseudoephedrine hydrochloride, 287*

Pseudo-Gest*
see *Pseudoephedrine hydrochloride, 287*

Q, R

Q-vel Soft Caplets*
see *Quinine sulfate, 31*

Quick Pep*
see *Caffeine, 30*

Quinalan*
see *Quinidine, 29*

Quinamm*
see *Quinine sulfate, 31*

Quinidex Extentabs*
see *Quinidine, 29*

Quinora*
see *Quinidine, 29*

Quiphile*
see *Quinine sulfate, 31*

Reglan*
see *Metoclopramide, 235*

Regular Insulin*
see *Insulin, 215*

Restoril*
see *Temazepam, 29*

Retrovir
see *Zidovudine, 341*

Rhindecon
see *Phenylpropanolamine hydrochloride, 268*

Rifadin*
see *Rifampin, 294*

Rimactane*
see *Rifampin, 294*

Ritalin
see *Methylphenidate hydrochloride, 233*

Ritalin-SR
see *Methylphenidate hydrochloride, 233*

Robaxin*
see *Methocarbamol, 30*

Robaxin-750*
see Methocarbamol, 30

Robicillin VK*
see Penicillin V potassium, 262

Robimycin*
see Erythromycin base, 165

Robitussin
see Guaifenesin, 195

Robitussin Cough Calmers
see Dextromethorphan, 144

Robitussin Pediatric
see Dextromethorphan, 144

Roxicodone*
see Oxycodone, 31

Roxicodone Intensol*
see Oxycodone, 31

S

Sandimmune*
see Cyclosporine, 131

Scabene*
see Lindane, 226

Scot-Tussin DM
see Dextromethorphan, 144

Scot-tussin Expectorant
see Guaifenesin, 195

Seconal sodium pulvules*
see Secobarbital sodium, 31

Sectral*
see Acebutolol, 29

Seldane
see Terfenadine, 309

Senexon*
see Senna, 31

Senolax*
see Senna, 31

Septra
see Trimethoprim with Sulfamethoxazole, 332

Septra DS
see Trimethoprim with Sulfamethoxazole, 332

Serax*
see Oxazepam, 31

Serentil*
see Mesoridazine, 29

Seromycin Pulvules*
see Cycloserine, 30

Simron
see Ferrous gluconate, 181

Sinequan*
see Doxepin, 29

Sinustop Pro*
see Pseudoephedrine hydrochloride, 287

Slo-bid Gyrocaps*
see Theophylline, 315

Slo-Phyllin*
see Theophylline, 315

Slo-Phyllin Gyrocaps*
see Theophylline, 315

Slow Fe
see Ferrous sulfate, 183

Sofarin*
see Warfarin sodium, 336

Solfoton*
see Phenobarbital, 266

Soriatane*
see Acitretin, 30

Spancap No. 1
see Dextroamphetamine, 142

Stelazine
see Trifluoperazine hydrochloride, 329

Sterapred*
see Prednisone, 275

Sterapred DS*
see Prednisone, 275

St. Joseph Aspirin-Free*
see Acetaminophen, 48

St. Joseph Cough Suppressant
see Dextromethorphan, 144

Stimate*
see Desmopressin, 30

Sucrets Cough Control
see Dextromethorphan, 144

Sudafed*
see Pseudoephedrine hydrochloride, 287

Sudafed 12 hours*
see Pseudoephedrine hydrochloride, 287

Sultrin*
see Sulfathiazole, 31

Sumycin*
see Tetracycline hydrochloride, 311

Suppap-120*
see Acetaminophen, 48

Suppap-325*
see Acetaminophen, 48

Suppap-650*
see Acetaminophen, 48

Suprax
see Cefixime, 93

Symadine
see Amantadine hydrochloride, 57

Symmetrel
see Amantadine hydrochloride, 57

Synacort
see Hydrocortisone, 204

Synthroid
see Levothyroxine sodium, 224

T

Tagamet*
see *Cimetidine, 111*

Tambocor*
see *Flecainide, 30*

Tapazole*
see *Methimazole, 30*

Taractan*
see *Chlorprothixene, 29*

Tavist*
see *Clemastine fumarate, 29*

Tavist-1*
see *Clemastine fumerate, 29*

Tegopen
see *Cloxacillin sodium, 124*

Tegretol*
see *Carbamazepine, 86*

Tegrin-HC
see *Hydrocortisone, 204*

Telachlor
see *Chlorpheniramine maleate, 105*

Tempra*
see *Acetaminophen, 48*

Tenormin*
see *Atenolol, 72*

Tetracap*
see *Tetracycline hydrochloride, 311*

Tetralan*
see *Tetracycline hydrochloride, 311*

Tetram*
see *Tetracycline hydrochloride, 311*

Thalitone*
see *Chlorthalidone, 30*

Theo-24*
see *Theophylline, 315*

Theobid Duracaps*
see *Theophylline, 315*

Theobid Jr. Duracaps*
see *Theophylline, 315*

Theoclear-80*
see *Theophylline, 315*

Theoclear L.A. *
see *Theophylline, 315*

Theo-Dur*
see *Theophylline, 315*

Theo-Dur Sprinkle*
see *Theophylline, 315*

Theolair*
see *Theophylline, 315*

Theolair-SR*
see *Theophylline, 315*

Thioridazine HCl
see *Thioridazine hydrochloride, 318*

Thioridazine HCl Intensol
see *Thioridazine hydrochloride, 318*

Thorazine*
see *Chlorpromazine hydrochloride, 108*

Thorazine Spansules*
see *Chlorpromazine hydrochloride, 108*

Thyro-Block*
see *Iodine, 29*

Tirend*
see *Caffeine, 30*

TMP-SMZ
see *Trimethoprim with Sulfamethoxazole, 332*

Tofranil*
see *Imipramine hydrochloride, 210*

Tofranil-PM*
see *Imipramine hydrochloride, 210*

Tolectin DS*
see *Tolmetin, 31*

Tolectin 600*
see *Tolmetin, 31*

Tolectin 200*
see *Tolmetin, 31*

Tonocard*
see *Tocainide, 31*

Topicycline
see *Tetracycline hydrochloride, 311*

Toprol XL*
see *Metoprolol, 29*

Toradol*
see *Ketorolac, 30*

Totacillin*
see *Ampicillin, 68*

Trandate*
see *Labetalol, 29*

Transderm-Scop*
see *Scopolamine, 31*

Trental*
see *Pentoxifylline, 31*

Triacet
see *Triamcinolone, 326*

Triderm
see *Triamcinolone, 326*

Trilafon*
see *Perphenazine, 29*

Trimox*
see *Amoxicillin, 62*

Trimpex*
see *Trimethoprim, 31*

Tusscapine*
see *Noscapine, 31*

Tusstat
see *Diphenhydramine hydrochloride, 154*

Tylenol*
see *Acetaminophen, 48*

Tylenol with Codeine
see *Acetaminophen with Codeine, 50*

U-Z

Ultracef*
see *Cefadroxil, 91*

Ultralente U*
see *Insulin, 215*

Ultrase MT20
see *Pancrelipase, 256*

Ultrase MT24
see *Pancrelipase, 256*

Uni-tussin
see *Guaifenesin, 195*

Unipen
see *Nafcillin sodium, 242*

Urecholine
see *Bethanechol chloride, 80*

Urobak
see *Sulfamethoxazole, 303*

Valium*
see *Diazepam, 29*

Valrelease*
see *Diazepam, 29*

Vancenase
see *Beclomethasone, 76*

Vancenase AQ
see *Beclomethasone, 76*

Vanceril
see *Beclomethasone, 76*

Vantin
see *Cefpodoxime proxetil, 95*

Vaponefrin
see *Epinephrine, 163*

Vasotec*
see *Enalapril maleate, 161*

V-cillin K*
see *Penicillin V potassium, 262*

Veetids*
see *Penicillin V potassium, 262*

Velosef*
see *Cephradine, 103*

Velosulin Human*
see *Insulin, 215*

Veltane
see *Brompheniramine maleate, 82*

Ventolin
see *Albuterol, 54*

Ventolin Rotacaps
see *Albuterol, 54*

Verelan*
see *Verapamil, 31*

Vibra-Tabs*
see *Doxycycline, 158*

Vibramycin*
see *Doxycycline, 158*

Vicks Formula 44
see *Dextromethorphan, 144*

Vicks Formula 44 Pediatric Formula
see *Dextromethorphan, 144*

Videx
see *Didanosine, 148*

Viokase
see *Pancrelipase, 256*

Vitamin B$_1$*
see *Thiamine, 31*

Vitamin B$_2$*
see *Riboflavin, 31*

Vitamin B$_6$*
see *Pyridoxine, 31*

Vitamin B$_{12}$*
see *Cyanocobalamin, 30*

Vitamin K*
see *Phytonadione, 31*

Vivarin*
see *Caffeine, 30*

Wymox*
see *Amoxicillin, 62*

Xanax*
see *Alprazolam, 29*

Zantac*
see *Ranitidine, 292*

Zarontin*
see *Ethosuximide, 177*

Zithromax
see *Azithromycin, 74*

Zovirax*
see *Acyclovir, 52*

Zyloprim*
see *Allopurinol, 30*

Zymase
see *Pancrelipase, 256*

MEDICATION PROFILES:

GENERIC NAMES,

BRAND NAMES,

COMMON USES,

USUAL DOSES,

MEDICATION INTERACTIONS,

ADVERSE SIDE EFFECTS,

STORAGE AND ADMINISTRATION,

AND

SPECIAL INSTRUCTIONS

A cetaminophen

Brand Names

Acephen
(rectal
suppository)

Acetaminophen
Uniserts
(rectal
suppository)

Anacin–3
(tablet)

Children's
Anacin–3
(chewable
tablet, liquid)

Children's
Feverall
(rectal
suppository)

Children's
Panadol
(chewable
tablet, liquid)

Children's
Tylenol
(chewable
tablet, liquid)

(continued next page)

Common Uses

Acetaminophen is a medicine used to relieve fever and mild-to-moderate pain. It blocks the production of chemicals in the brain responsible for pain and also affects the temperature-regulating center of the brain. Acetaminophen does not relieve inflammation. Therefore, it may not relieve all the pain due to arthritis or other joint or tissue inflammatory disease.

Usual Dose

TABLET, CHEWABLE TABLET, CAPSULE, AND LIQUID

Children younger than 12 years: 10–15 mg/kg/dose given every 4–6 hours as needed for pain or fever. Maximum dose 5 g/day.

Children older than 12 years and Adults: 325–650 mg/dose given every 4–6 hours or 1000 mg dose every 6–8 hours as needed for pain or fever. Maximum dose 4 g/day.

RECTAL SUPPOSITORY

See the Medication Administration section for instructions on the proper use of a rectal suppository (page 18).

Children 3–6 years old: 120 mg/dose given every 4–6 hours as needed for fever. Maximum dose 720 mg/day.

Children 6–12 years old: 325 mg/dose given every 4–6 hours as needed for fever. Maximum dose 2600 mg/day.

Adults: 650 mg/dose given every 4–6 hours as needed for fever. Maximum of 6 doses a day.

Medication Interactions

Acetaminophen may decrease the effectiveness of:

rimantadine

Medications that increase the risk for the development of liver toxicity when combined with acetaminophen are:

alcohol

phenytoin

sulfinpyrazone

Adverse Side Effects

Minor: Dizziness, trembling.

Severe: Fatigue, rash, hives, sore throat, fever, blood in the urine, unusual bruising or bleeding, yellow skin or eyes.

Storage and Administration

The oral medicine should be stored in a cool, dry place away from light. Prolonged exposure to heat, moisture, or light can damage the medicine.

The liquid may be stored at room temperature and does not need to be refrigerated.

Refrigeration of the rectal suppositories is recommended.

If upset stomach occurs, the medicine can be given with food.

The chewable tablet should be chewed thoroughly before swallowing.

If the child is unable to swallow pills, the nonchewable tablets can be crushed or the capsules opened and mixed with a small amount of water or soft food (such as applesauce, pudding, jam, or jelly). This mixture should be swallowed and not chewed. The entire mixture must be swallowed to ensure that the child received the full dose.

Even though liquid acetaminophen does not taste bad, some children may not want to take it. If this occurs, the liquid medicine can be disguised by mixing the dose with water or juice. The entire mixture must be swallowed to ensure that the child received the full dose.

Special Instructions

The child's physician should be notified if the pain or fever is not relieved by the medicine.

Brand Names

(continued)

Junior Strength
  Feverall
  (rectal
  suppository)

Neopap
  (rectal
  suppository)

Panadol
  (tablet)

St. Joseph
  Aspirin-Free
  (chewable
  tablet, liquid)

Suppap-120
  (rectal
  suppository)

Suppap-325
  (rectal
  suppository)

Suppap-650
  (rectal
  suppository)

Tempra
  (chewable
  tablet, liquid)

Tylenol
  (capsule,
  tablet, liquid)

Acetaminophen with Codeine

Brand Names

Capital with
  Codeine
  (liquid)
Phenaphen
  with Codeine
  (tablet,
  capsule)
Tylenol with
  Codeine
  (tablet, liquid)

Common Uses

Acetaminophen with codeine is a combination medicine used to relieve mild-to-severe pain. The acetaminophen portion relieves pain by blocking the production of chemicals in the brain responsible for pain. The codeine portion relieves pain by binding to specific chemical receptors that relieve pain. These medicines work together to provide better pain relief than either one alone.

Usual Dose

Children: 0.5–1 mg of codeine/kg/dose given every 4–6 hours.

Adults: 1–2 tablets given every 4 hours. Maximum dose 12 tablets/day.

Medication Interactions

Acetaminophen with codeine may decrease the effectiveness of:

rimantadine

Medications that increase the risk for the development of liver toxicity when combined with acetaminophen with codeine are:

alcohol

phenytoin

sulfinpyrazone

Adverse Side Effects

Minor: Nausea, constipation, dizziness, drowsiness, sedation, dry mouth, sweating.

Severe: Difficulty breathing, excitation, awareness of heartbeat, fever, sore throat.

Storage and Administration

The oral medicine should be stored in a cool, dry place away from light. Prolonged exposure to heat, moisture, or light can damage the medicine.

The liquid may be stored at room temperature and does not need to be refrigerated.

If the child is unable to swallow pills, the tablets can be crushed or the capsules opened and mixed with a small amount of water or soft food (such as applesauce, pudding, jam, or jelly). This mixture should be swallowed and not chewed. The entire mixture must be swallowed to ensure that the child received the full dose.

If upset stomach occurs, the medicine can be given with food.

Special Instructions

May cause sedation, drowsiness, and dizziness in some people. Until it is known how the child will react to the medicine, activities that require mental alertness (such as physical education and playground activity) should be restricted.

May cause dizziness upon standing; therefore, always have the child stand up slowly. If the child becomes dizzy, he should be instructed to sit or lie down immediately.

For older children, dry mouth may be relieved by chewing gum or sucking on hard candy or ice chips. Younger children may need extra liquids.

N o t e s

A cyclovir

Brand Name

Zovirax
(tablet,
capsule,
liquid,
skin ointment)

Common Uses

Acyclovir belongs to the class of medicines called anti-virals. Acyclovir is effective in treating and preventing various viral infections caused by herpesvirus and vari-cella-zoster virus by preventing the viruses from growing.

Acyclovir is not effective in treating infections caused by bacteria, parasites, or yeast.

Usual Dose

HERPESVIRUS

Children: 250–600 mg/m²/dose given 4–5 times a day.

Adults: 800 mg/dose given 5 times a day.

VARICELLA-ZOSTER VIRUS

Children: 10–20 mg/kg/dose given 4 times a day. Maximum dose 800 mg/dose.

Adults: 20 mg/kg/dose given 4–5 times a day (maximum dose 800 mg/dose), 600–800 mg/dose given 5 times a day, or 1000 mg/dose given every 6 hours.

SKIN OINTMENT

Children and Adults: Apply as directed to the infect-ed area(s) 6 times a day.

Medication Interactions

No major medication interactions have been found with other oral medications.

Adverse Side Effects

Minor

TABLET, CAPSULE, AND LIQUID: Nausea, diarrhea, upset stomach, constipation, dizziness, headache.

SKIN MEDICINE: Acne, dry skin, mild burning or stinging sensation, itching, minor rash.

Severe: Severe nausea or diarrhea, stomach pain, vomiting, painful urination, blood in the urine, decrease in frequency of urination, sore throat, fever, rash, hives, skin blistering, severe or persistent skin irritation, leg or joint pain, muscle cramps, fast heartbeat, depression, fatigue, confusion, hallucinations, insomnia, loss of appetite, seizures, unusual bruising or bleeding, yellow skin or eyes, difficulty breathing.

Storage and Administration

The oral medicine should be stored in a cool, dry place away from light. Prolonged exposure to heat, moisture, or light can damage the medicine.

Before measuring the dose, the liquid form of this medicine should be shaken well. The liquid may be stored at room temperature and does not need to be refrigerated.

The skin ointment may be stored at room temperature.

Acyclovir should be taken with food or milk to decrease or prevent stomach upset.

It is best for the child to take this medicine with a full glass of water and drink plenty of water between doses.

If the child is unable to swallow pills, the tablets can be crushed or the capsules opened and mixed with water or soft food (such as apple-sauce, pudding, jam, or jelly). This mixture then should be swallowed and not chewed. The entire mixture must be taken to ensure that the child received the entire dose.

Special Instructions

Acyclovir may cause dizziness in some people. Until it is known how the child will react to the medicine, activities that require mental alertness (such as physical education and playground activity) should be restricted.

Skin medicine is to be used only on the skin. Be careful not to get it into the child's eyes.

N o t e s

A lbuterol

Brand Names

Proventil
(tablet, liquid,
oral inhaler,
solution for
inhalation)

Proventil
Repetabs
(long-acting
tablet)

Ventolin
(tablet, liquid,
oral inhaler,
solution for
inhalation)

Ventolin
Rotacaps
(capsule for
inhalation)

Common Uses

Albuterol belongs to the class of medicines called bronchodilators, which are used to treat and prevent asthma attacks and lessen breathing difficulties caused by various other non–infection-related respiratory problems. Albuterol is effective by opening the airways and then preventing them from closing again.

Usual Dose

SYRUP

Children 2–6 years old: 0.1–0.2 mg/kg/dose given 3 times a day. Maximum dose 12 mg/day.

Children 6–14 years old: 2 mg/dose given 3–4 times a day. Maximum dose 24 mg/day.

Children older than 14 years and Adults: 2–4 mg/dose given 3–4 times a day. Maximum dose 32 mg/day.

TABLETS

Children 6–12 years old: 2 mg/dose given 3–4 times a day. Maximum dose 24 mg/day.

Children 12 years or older and Adults: 2–4 mg/dose given 3–4 times a day. The usual dose of long-acting tablets is 4–8 mg/dose every 12 hours. Maximum dose 32 mg/day.

ORAL INHALATION

See the Medication Administration section for instructions on the proper use of an oral inhaler (page 10).

Children younger than 12 years: 1–2 puffs given 4 times a day.

Children 12 years or older and Adults: 1–2 puffs given every 4–6 hours.

SOLUTION FOR INHALATION

See the Medication Administration section for instructions on the proper use of a nebulizer (page 13).

Infants: 0.05–0.15 mg/kg/dose given every 4–6 hours.

Children younger than 12 years: 1.25–2.5 mg/dose given every 4–6 hours.

Children 12 years or older and Adults: 2.5 mg/dose given every 6–8 hours.

Note: There are 2 concentrations of albuterol available. The 0.5% solution must be diluted with normal saline; 0.5 mL of this solution provides 2.5 mg of albuterol. The 0.083% solution does not need to be diluted; 3 mL of this solution provides 2.5 mg of albuterol.

CAPSULES FOR INHALATION

See the Medication Administration section for instructions on the proper use of a Rotahaler (page 12).

Children older than 4 years and Adults: 1–2 capsules/dose given every 4–6 hours.

Medication Interactions

No major medication interactions have been found with other oral medications.

Adverse Side Effects

Minor

ORAL INHALATION: Dry throat and mouth. Side effects listed in the Solution for Inhalation section (below) can also occur when too many inhalations are given or when the medicine is given too often.

SOLUTION FOR INHALATION: Dry throat and mouth, nervousness, headache, fast heartbeat, trembling, dizziness, flushing.

CAPSULES FOR INHALATION: Coughing, dry throat and mouth. Side effects listed under the Solution for Inhalation section (above) can also occur when too many capsules are given or when the medicine is given too often.

TABLETS AND SYRUP: Nervousness, headache, fast heartbeat, trembling, insomnia, increased blood pressure, dizziness, drowsiness, nausea, vomiting, hyperactivity, flushing, upset stomach.

Children may be more susceptible to side effects of insomnia, nervousness, hyperactivity, and fast heartbeat than adults.

Severe: Chest pain, hallucinations, difficult or painful urination, rash, irregular heartbeat.

A

Storage and Administration

The oral medicine should be stored in a cool, dry place away from light. Prolonged exposure to heat, moisture, or light can damage the medicine.

The liquid may be stored at room temperature and does not need to be refrigerated.

The inhaler should be kept in a cool place. Do not puncture or expose the inhaler to prolonged periods of heat.

The solution and capsules for inhalation should be stored in a cool, dry place away from light. Prolonged exposure to heat, moisture, or light can damage the medicine.

Best if taken on an empty stomach (1 hour before a meal or 2–3 hours after a meal). However, if the child develops an upset stomach from albuterol, it can be given with food or milk.

The long-acting tablet should be swallowed whole with a full glass of water. Do not crush or allow the child to chew it.

If the child is unable to swallow the non–long-acting tablets, they can be crushed and mixed with a small amount of water or soft food (such as applesauce, pudding, jam, or jelly). This mixture should be swallowed and not chewed. The entire mixture must be swallowed to ensure that the child received the full dose.

For proper use of the oral and capsule inhaler and nebulizer read the appropriate medication administration section (pages 10–13).

To prevent dry throat and mouth, have the child rinse her mouth with water after each inhalation.

If the child is receiving more than one puff of the oral inhaler, give the second puff at least 1 minute after first one.

If the child is receiving another inhaled medicine for asthma, the entire inhaled albuterol dose should be given at least 10–15 minutes before the other inhaled medicine is given, or as directed by the physician.

Special Instructions

May cause dizziness or drowsiness in some people. Until it is known how the child will react to the medicine, activities that require mental alertness (such as physical education and playground activity) should be restricted.

Consult the child's physician about giving extra inhalations, because increasing the number of inhalations may be dangerous.

Have the child avoid eating excessive amounts of chocolate and drinking beverages containing caffeine; these may make her more susceptible to insomnia, irritability, and hyperactivity.

For older children, dry mouth may be relieved by chewing gum or sucking on hard candy or ice chips. Younger children may need extra liquids.

Amantadine hydrochloride

Common Uses

Amantadine belongs to the class of medicines called antivirals. Amantadine is prescribed for viral infections of the respiratory tract caused by influenza. It is effective against these infections because it prevents the virus from growing.

Amantadine is not effective against infections caused by other viruses, bacteria, parasites, or yeast.

Usual Dose

TREATMENT

Children 1–8 years old: 4.4–8.8 mg/kg/day divided into equal doses given 1–2 times a day. Maximum dose 150 mg/day.

Children 9–12 years old: 100–200 mg/day divided into equal doses given 1–2 times a day.

Children older than 12 years and Adults: 200 mg/day divided into equal doses given 1–2 times a day.

PREVENTION

Amantadine is started after the child has been exposed to influenza and is continued for 10 days.

Medication Interactions

No major medication interactions have been found with other oral medications.

Adverse Side Effects

Minor: Nausea, vomiting, constipation, dizziness, dry mouth, headache, insomnia, loss of appetite, difficulty concentrating, fatigue.

Severe: Anxiety, depression, hallucinations, seizures, difficulty breathing, fever, sore throat, vision changes, uncontrolled rolling of the eyes, rash, purple-red spots on the skin, fainting, slurred speech, difficult or painful urination, irregular heartbeat.

Brand Names

Symadine
(capsule)
Symmetrel
(capsule,
liquid)

A

Storage and Administration

The oral medicine should be stored in a cool, dry place away from light. Prolonged exposure to heat, moisture, or light can damage the medicine.

The liquid may be stored at room temperature and does not need to be refrigerated.

If upset stomach occurs, the medicine can be given with food or milk.

If the child is unable to swallow the capsules, they can be opened and mixed with a small amount of water or soft food (such as applesauce, pudding, jam, or jelly). This mixture should be swallowed and not chewed. The entire mixture must be swallowed to ensure that the child received the full dose.

Special Instructions

May cause dizziness in some people. Until it is known how the child will react to the medicine, activities that require mental alertness (such as physical education and playground activity) should be restricted.

May cause dizziness upon standing; therefore, always have the child stand up slowly. If the child becomes dizzy, he should be instructed to sit or lie down immediately.

In children with a seizure disorder, this medicine may cause seizures even if the seizures are currently controlled.

For older children, dry mouth may be relieved by chewing gum or sucking on hard candy or ice chips. Younger children may need extra liquids.

N o t e s

Amitriptyline hydrochloride

Common Uses

Amitriptyline belongs to the class of medicines called tricyclic antidepressants. Amitriptyline is used to treat various forms of depression by increasing the concentration of chemicals in the brain that help counteract the depression. Amitriptyline also can be used to treat certain types of chronic pain and nerve pain.

Usual Dose

Children: 0.1–2 mg/kg given at bedtime. Start with the lowest dose and increase according to the physician's directions.

Adolescents: 25–100 mg/day divided into equal doses given 1–4 times a day. Start with the lowest dose and increase according to the physician's directions.

Adults: 30–300 mg/day divided into equal doses given 1–4 times a day.

Medication Interactions

Medications that increase the risk for the development of amitriptyline adverse side effects are:

    cimetidine

    fluoxetine

Amitriptyline decreases the effectiveness of:

    clonidine

    guanethidine

Amitriptyline increases the risk for the development of bleeding with:

    dicumarol

Medications that may cause seizures, dangerous increases in body temperature, sweating, headache, fast heartbeat, or death when combined with amitriptyline are:

    isocarboxazid

    phenelzine

    tranylcypromine

Brand Names

Elavil
  (tablet)
Endep
  (tablet)

A

Medications that may increase the risk of sedation, drowsiness, and dizziness when combined with amitriptyline are:

bromphenaramine

chlorpheniramine

diphenhydramine

Adverse Side Effects

Minor: Sedation, drowsiness, insomnia, dry mouth, constipation, fatigue, bad taste in mouth, blurred vision, dizziness, increased sensitivity to sunlight, nervousness, anxiety, sweating, nausea, vomiting, blue-green urine.

Severe: Confusion; seizures; chest pain; fever; sore throat; hallucinations; irregular heartbeat; stomach pain; loss of balance; unusual bruising or bleeding; yellow skin or eyes; joint pain; swollen breasts; trembling; unintentional movements of face, mouth, and tongue.

Storage and Administration

Amitriptyline should be stored in a cool, dry place away from light. Prolonged exposure to heat, moisture, or light can damage the medicine.

Best if taken on an empty stomach (1 hour before a meal or 2–3 hours after a meal). However, if amitriptyline upsets the child's stomach, it can be given with food or milk.

If the child is unable to swallow the tablets, they can be crushed and mixed with a small amount of water or soft food (such as applesauce, pudding, jam, or jelly). This mixture should be swallowed and not chewed. The entire mixture must be swallowed to ensure that the child received the full dose.

Special Instructions

May cause sedation, drowsiness, and dizziness in some people. Until it is known how the child will react to the medicine, activities that require mental alertness (such as physical education and playground activity) should be restricted.

May cause dizziness upon standing; therefore, always have the child stand up slowly. If she becomes dizzy, she should be instructed to sit or lie down immediately.

In children with a seizure disorder, this medicine may cause seizures even if the seizures are currently controlled.

May cause the urine to become blue-green in color. This effect occurs often and is harmless.

For older children, dry mouth may be relieved by chewing gum or sucking on hard candy or ice chips. Younger children may need extra liquids.

Amitriptyline may cause the child to become more sensitive to sunlight; therefore, prolonged exposure to sunlight should be avoided.

The child should not abruptly stop taking this medicine. Suddenly stopping the medicine can cause nausea, headache, upset stomach, fatigue, or depression.

N o t e s

A moxicillin

Brand Names

Amoxil
  (chewable
  tablet,
  capsule,
  liquid)
Biomox
  (capsule,
  liquid)
Polymox
  (capsule,
  liquid)
Trimox
  (capsule,
  liquid)
Wymox
  (capsule,
  liquid)

Common Uses

Amoxicillin belongs to the class of medicines called antibiotics, which are used to treat a variety of bacterial infections. Amoxicillin is prescribed for infections of the middle ear, respiratory tract, urinary tract, and skin, because it prevents the bacteria from growing.

Amoxicillin is effective only against bacterial infections, not those caused by viruses, parasites, or yeast.

Usual Dose

Children: 20–50 mg/kg/day divided into equal doses given every 8 hours. A child weighing more than 20 kg (44 lb) may be given the adult dose.

Adults: 250–500 mg/dose given every 8 hours. Maximum dose 2–3 g/day.

Medication Interactions

Medications that decrease the effectiveness of amoxicillin are:

demeclocycline	minocycline
doxycycline	oxytetracycline
methacycline	tetracycline

Adverse Side Effects

Minor: Diarrhea, nausea, vomiting, heartburn, upset stomach, darkened tongue.

Severe: Rash, hives, difficulty breathing, blood in the urine, sore throat, fever, stomach cramps, seizures, unexplained bleeding or bruising, severe diarrhea.

Storage and Administration

The oral medicine should be stored in a cool, dry place away from light. Prolonged exposure to heat, moisture, or light can damage the medicine.

Before measuring the dose, the liquid form of amoxicillin should be shaken well. Refrigeration of the liquid is recommended. After receiving the liquid medicine

A

from the pharmacy, it is good only for 14 days; therefore, always check the expiration date on the prescription label before using.

If upset stomach occurs, the medicine can be given with food or milk.

The chewable tablet should be chewed thoroughly before swallowing.

If the child is unable to swallow the capsule, it can be opened and mixed with water, fruit juice, carbonated beverage, or soft food (such as applesauce, pudding, jam, or jelly). This mixture should be swallowed and not chewed. The entire mixture must be swallowed to ensure that the child received the full dose.

Special Instructions

The child's physician should be notified if the infection worsens or does not improve within 3–5 days.

The child's physician should be notified if a rash develops while she is taking amoxicillin.

N o t e s

A moxicillin and Clavulanic acid

Brand Names

Augmentin
(tablet,
chewable
tablet, liquid)

Common Uses

The amoxicillin and clavulanic acid combination belongs to the class of medicine called antibiotics, which are used to treat a variety of bacterial infections. It is prescribed for infections of the middle ear, respiratory tract, urinary tract, and skin, and works by preventing the bacteria from growing.

The amoxicillin and clavulanic acid combination is effective only against bacterial infections, not those caused by viruses, parasites, or yeast.

Usual Dose

Children 40 kg (88 lb) or less: 20–40 mg/kg/day of amoxicillin divided into equal doses given every 8 hours. Children who weigh more than 40 kg may be given the adult dose.

Children weighing more than 40 kg and Adults: 250–500 mg/dose given every 8 hours. Maximum dose 2 g/day.

Medication Interactions

Medications that decrease the effectiveness of the amoxicillin and clavulanic acid combination are:

demeclocycline	minocycline
doxycycline	oxytetracycline
methacycline	tetracycline

Adverse Side Effects

Minor: Diarrhea, nausea, vomiting, heartburn, upset stomach, darkened tongue.

Severe: Rash, hives, difficulty breathing, blood in the urine, sore throat, fever, stomach cramps, seizures, unexplained bleeding or bruising, severe diarrhea.

Storage and Administration

The oral medicine should be stored in a cool, dry

place away from light. Prolonged exposure to heat, moisture, or light can damage the medicine.

Before measuring the dose of the liquid form of amoxicillin and clavulanic acid, it should be shaken well. Refrigeration of the liquid is recommended. After receiving the liquid medicine from the pharmacy, it is good only for 10 days; therefore, always check the expiration date on the prescription label before using.

If upset stomach occurs, the medicine can be given with food.

The chewable tablet should be chewed thoroughly before swallowing.

If the child is unable to swallow the nonchewable tablet, it can be crushed and mixed with water, fruit juice, carbonated beverage, or soft food (such as applesauce, pudding, jam, or jelly). This mixture should be swallowed and not chewed. The entire mixture must be swallowed to ensure that the child received the entire dose.

Special Instructions

The child's physician should be notified if the infection worsens or does not improve within 3–5 days.

The child's physician should be notified if a rash develops while he is taking this medicine.

N o t e s

A mphetamine

Brand Name

None
Generic
  medicine
  dosage form:
Amphetamine
(tablet)

Common Uses

Amphetamine belongs to the class of medicines called stimulants. Amphetamine is used to treat narcolepsy and attention deficit disorder with hyperactivity (ADDH). Amphetamine is able to treat these conditions, causing certain chemicals to be released into the brain, which allows more focused attention.

Usual Dose

NARCOLEPSY

Children 6–12 years old: Start with 5 mg/day and increase the dose according to the physician's directions until the desired effect is obtained. Maximum dose 60 mg/day.

Children older than 12 years and Adults: Start with 10 mg/day and increase the dose according to the physician's directions until the desired effect is obtained.

ATTENTION DEFICIT DISORDER WITH HYPERACTIVITY

Children 3–5 years old: Start with 2.5 mg/dose given in the morning. Adjust the dose according to the physician's directions until the desired effect is obtained. Maximum dose 40 mg/day.

Children age 6 or older: Start with 5 mg/dose given 1–2 times a day. Adjust the dose according to the physician's directions until the desired effect is obtained. Maximum dose 40 mg/day.

Medication Interactions

Medications that increase the risk for the development of amphetamine adverse side effects are:

furazolidone	sodium bicarbonate
potassium citrate	sodium citrate
sodium acetate	sodium lactate

Amphetamine decreases the effectiveness of:

guanethidine

Medications that may cause dangerous increases in body temperature, brain hemorrhage, seizures, or death when combined with amphetamine are:

isocarboxazid   phenelzine

pargyline   tranylcypromine

Adverse Side Effects

Minor: Constipation, nausea, diarrhea, dizziness, dry mouth, insomnia, irritability, loss of appetite, hyperactivity, bad taste in mouth, upset stomach, nervousness.

Severe: Blurred vision; confusion; fatigue; headache; awareness of heartbeat; rapid heartbeat; rash; sweating; chest pain; trembling; hives; uncontrolled movements of head, arms, or legs.

Storage and Administration

The oral medicine should be stored in a cool, dry place away from light. Prolonged exposure to heat, moisture, or light can damage the medicine. The tablet should not be crushed and mixed for administration.

It is best to take amphetamine with food or milk to decrease or prevent stomach upset.

Special Instructions

May cause dizziness in some people. Until it is known how the child will react to the medicine, activities that require mental alertness (such as physical education and playground activity) should be restricted.

For older children, dry mouth may be relieved by chewing gum or sucking on hard candy or ice chips. Younger children may need extra liquids.

Have the child avoid drinking beverage containing caffeine and eating excessive amounts of chocolate—these may make him susceptible to insomnia, irritability, and hyperactivity.

A mpicillin

Omnipen
(capsule,
liquid)
Polycillin
(capsule,
liquid)
Principen
(capsule,
liquid)
Totacillin
(capsule,
liquid)

Common Uses

Ampicillin belongs to the class of medicines called antibiotics, which are used to treat a variety of bacterial infections. Ampicillin is prescribed for infections of the middle ear, respiratory tract, and urinary tract, because it prevents the bacteria from growing.

Ampicillin is effective only against bacterial infections, not those caused by viruses, parasites, or yeast.

Usual Dose

Children: 50–100 mg/kg/day divided into equal doses given every 6 hours. Maximum dose 2–3 g/day.

Adults: 250–500 mg/dose given every 6 hours.

Medication Interactions

Medications that decrease the effectiveness of ampicillin are:

demeclocycline	minocycline
doxycycline	oxytetracycline
methacycline	tetracycline

Ampicillin decreases the effectiveness of:

atenolol

A medication that increases the risk for the development of skin rash when combined with ampicillin is:

allopurinol

Adverse Side Effects

Minor: Diarrhea occurs more often with ampicillin than with other antibiotics. Other side effects include nausea, vomiting, heartburn, upset stomach, darkened tongue.

Severe: Rash, hives, difficulty breathing, blood in the urine, sore throat, fever, stomach cramps, seizures, unexplained bleeding or bruising, severe diarrhea.

Storage and Administration

The medicine should be stored in a cool, dry place away from light. Prolonged exposure to heat, moisture, or light can damage the medicine.

Before measuring the dose, the liquid form of ampicillin should be shaken well. Refrigeration of the liquid is recommended. After receiving the liquid medicine from the pharmacy, it is good only for 14 days; therefore, always check the expiration date on the prescription label before using.

If the child is unable to swallow capsules, they can be opened and mixed with a small amount of water. The entire mixture must be swallowed to ensure that the child received the full dose.

Should be taken on an empty stomach (1 hour before a meal or 2–3 hours after a meal).

Special Instructions

The child's physician should be notified if the infection worsens or does not improve within 3–5 days.

The child's physician should be notified if a rash develops while she is taking this medicine.

N o t e s

A stemizole

Brand Name

Hismanal
(tablet)

Common Uses

Astemizole belongs to the class of medicines called antihistamines. Astemizole is used to treat seasonal and constant runny noses due to allergies by blocking the chemical histamine, which causes these problems.

Usual Dose

Children younger than 6 years: 0.2 mg/kg/dose given once a day.

Children 6–12 years old: 5 mg/dose given once a day.

Children older than 12 years and Adults: 10–30 mg/dose given once a day.

Medication Interactions

Medications that increase the risk for the development of astemizole adverse side effects are:

azithromycin   itraconazole

clarithromycin   ketoconazole

erythromycin   troleandomycin

fluconazole

Adverse Side Effects

Minor: Diarrhea; upset stomach; dry mouth, nose, or throat; dizziness; headache; increased appetite; weight gain; nervousness; increased sensitivity to sunlight.

Severe: Difficulty breathing, sore throat, rash, hair loss, tingling in hands or feet, muscle aches, yellow skin or eyes.

Storage and Administration

The oral medicine should be stored in a cool, dry place away from light. Prolonged exposure to heat, moisture, or light can damage the medicine.

Should be taken on an empty stomach (1 hour before a meal or 2–3 hours after a meal).

If the child is unable to swallow the astemizole tablet, it can be crushed and mixed with water. This mixture should be swallowed and not chewed. The entire mixture must be swallowed to ensure that the child received the full dose.

Special Instructions

May cause dizziness in some people. Until it is known how the child will react to the medicine, activities that require mental alertness (such as physical education and playground activity) should be restricted.

For older children, dry mouth may be relieved by chewing gum or sucking on hard candy or ice chips. Younger children may need extra liquids.

Have the child avoid prolonged exposure to sunlight; this medication causes the child to be more sensitive to it.

N o t e s

A tenolol

Tenormin
(tablet)

Common Uses

Atenolol belongs to the class of medicines called beta-blockers. Atenolol is used to treat and control high blood pressure and prevent chest pain, by blocking specific impulses that may cause or worsen these conditions.

Usual Dose

Children: 1–2 mg/kg/dose given once a day.

Adults: 50–100 mg/dose given once a day.

Medication Interactions

Medications that may decrease the effectiveness of atenolol are:

ampicillin   indomethacin

ibuprofen   piroxicam

Atenolol decreases the effectiveness of:

clonidine

A medication that may cause increased risk for dizziness upon standing when combined with atenolol is:

prazosin

Adverse Side Effects

Minor: Nausea; diarrhea; constipation; upset stomach; headache; dizziness; drowsiness; anxiety; nervousness; difficulty sleeping; dry eyes, mouth, or skin; fatigue; weakness, blurred vision.

Severe: Difficulty breathing, wheezing, slow heartbeat, chest pain, cold hands or feet, numbness or tingling of fingers or toes, swelling of legs or feet, joint pain, confusion, persistent dizziness, continued fatigue or weakness, persistent headache, reduced alertness, depression, rash, unusual bruising or bleeding, sudden weight gain, nightmares.

Storage and Administration

The oral medicine should be stored in a cool, dry place away from light. Prolonged exposure to heat, moisture, or light can damage the medicine.

If upset stomach occurs, atenolol can be given with food or milk.

If the child is unable to swallow the tablet, it can be crushed and mixed with water, juice, or soft food (such as applesauce, pudding, jam, or jelly). This mixture should be swallowed and not chewed. The entire mixture must be swallowed to ensure that the child received the entire dose.

Special Instructions

May cause drowsiness or dizziness in some people. Until it is known how the child will react to the medicine, activities that require mental alertness (such as physical education and playground activity) should be restricted.

May cause dizziness upon standing; therefore, always have the child stand up slowly. If the child becomes dizzy he should be instructed to sit or lie down immediately.

For older children, dry mouth may be relieved by chewing gum or sucking on hard candy or ice chips. Younger children may need extra liquids.

Dry eyes may be relieved by using artificial tears.

It is very important that this medicine is not suddenly stopped; this would cause the blood pressure to become very high.

N o t e s

A zithromycin

Common Uses

Azithromycin belongs to the class of medicines called antibiotics, which are used to treat a variety of bacterial infections. Azithromycin is prescribed for infections of the respiratory tract and skin, because it prevents the bacteria from growing.

Azithromycin is effective only against bacterial infections, not those caused by viruses, parasites, or yeast.

Usual Dose

Children younger than 16 years: 10 mg/kg/day given once a day on the first day and then 5 mg/kg/day given once a day for the next 4 days.

Children 16 years or older and Adults: 500 mg once a day given on the first day and then 250 mg/day given once a day for the next 4 days.

Medication Interactions

Medications that may decrease the effectiveness of azithromycin are:

antacids

Azithromycin increases the risk for the development of adverse side effects of:

astemizole   loratadine

carbamazepine   terfenadine

Adverse Side Effects

Minor: Nausea, vomiting, diarrhea, upset stomach, dizziness, drowsiness, fatigue, headache, rash, awareness of heartbeat, increased sensitivity to sunlight.

Severe: Stomach pain, dark urine, pale stools, itching, sore throat, fever, yellow skin or eyes, unusual bruising or bleeding.

Storage and Administration

The oral medicine should be stored in a cool, dry place away from light. Prolonged exposure to heat, moisture, or light can damage the medicine.

Should be taken on an empty stomach (1 hour before a meal or 2–3 hours after a meal).

If the child is unable to swallow the azithromycin capsule, it can be opened and mixed with a small amount of water. This mixture should be swallowed and not chewed. The entire mixture must be swallowed to ensure that the child received the full dose.

Do not give the child any antacids within 2 hours before and 2 hours after taking azithromycin.

Special Instructions

The child's physician should be notified if the infection worsens or does not improve within 2–3 days.

May cause dizziness or drowsiness in some people. Until it is known how the child will react to the medicine, activities that require mental alertness (such as physical education and playground activity) should be restricted.

Have the child avoid prolonged exposure to sunlight; this medication may cause the child to be more sensitive to it.

N o t e s

B eclomethasone

Brand Names

Beclovent
(oral inhaler)
Beconase
(nasal aerosol)
Beconase AQ
(nasal spray)
Vancenase
(nasal aerosol)
Vancenase AQ
(nasal spray)
Vanceril
(oral inhaler)

Common Uses

Beclomethasone belongs to the class of medicines called corticosteroids. Oral inhalation of the medicine is used to prevent asthma attacks. Nasal inhalation is used to provide relief of stuffy nose and nasal irritation and discomfort due to hay fever and allergies. Beclomethasone is able to be used in these conditions because it affects many different substances in the body that may cause or worsen these conditions.

Usual Dose

ORAL INHALATION: See the Medication Administration section for instructions on the proper use of an oral inhaler (page 10).

Children 6–12 years old: 1–2 inhalations 3–4 times a day. Maximum dose 10 inhalations/day.

Children older than 12 years and Adults: 2 inhalations 3–4 times a day or 2 sprays in each nostril twice a day. Maximum dose 20 inhalations/day.

NASAL INHALATION: See the Medication Administration section for instructions on the proper use of a nasal spray and aerosol spray (pages 15 and 16).

Children 6–12 years old: 1 spray in each nostril 3 times a day.

Children older than 12 years and Adults: 1 spray in each nostril 2–4 times a day.

Medication Interactions

No major medication interactions have been found with other oral medications.

Adverse Side Effects

Minor

ORAL INHALATION: Fungal growth in mouth, hoarseness, dry mouth, bad taste in mouth, cough, headache, dizziness.

NASAL INHALATION: Irritation and burning of nose, sneezing, fungal growth in nose, stuffy or runny nose, bad taste in mouth, headache, dizziness.

Severe: Rash, difficulty swallowing, hives, increased thirst.

Storage and Administration

The oral and nasal medicine should be kept in a cool place. Do not puncture or expose the oral inhaler or nasal aerosol to prolonged periods of heat.

For proper use of the oral or nasal medicine read the appropriate medication administration section.

Have the child gargle or rinse her mouth with water to prevent some of the adverse side effects associated with oral inhalation.

If the child is also using an orally inhaled bronchodilator (such as albuterol, metaproterenol, or terbutaline) give the entire bronchodilator dose at least 10–15 minutes, or as directed by a physician, before giving beclomethasone oral inhalations.

Special Instructions

Oral inhalation of beclomethasone is used to prevent asthma attacks, but it does not treat an asthma attack that is occurring. When one does occur this medicine will not help.

May cause dizziness in some children. Until it is known how the child will react to the medicine, activities that require mental alertness (such as physical education and playground activity) should be restricted.

N o t e s

Benztropine mesylate

Cogentin
(tablet)

Common Uses

Benztropine belongs to the class of medicines called anticholinergics. Benzotropine is used to alleviate uncontrolled shaking and trembling caused by certain diseases and medicine by balancing the amount of certain chemicals in the body.

Usual Dose

Children older than 3 years: 0.02–0.05 mg/kg/dose given 1–2 times a day.

Adults: 1–4 mg/dose given 1–2 times a day.

Medication Interactions

Benztropine may decrease the effectiveness of:

chlorpromazine	prochlorperazine
fluphenazine	promethazine
haloperidol	thioridazine
perphenazine	trifluoperazine

Adverse Side Effects

Minor: Nausea; vomiting; constipation; upset stomach; dizziness; drowsiness; blurred vision; dry eyes, throat, nose, and mouth; increased sensitivity of eyes to light; headache; nervousness; decreased sweating; difficult or painful urination.

Severe: Hallucinations, depression, mood changes, unusual restlessness, awareness of heartbeat, fast heartbeat, numbness or tingling in hands or feet, rash, difficulty breathing, seizures, persistent difficulty in urination, eye pain, memory loss, swollen neck glands.

B

Storage and Administration

The oral medicine should be stored in a cool, dry place away from light. Prolonged exposure to heat, moisture, or light can damage the medicine.

It is best to take benztropine mesylate with food or milk to decrease or prevent stomach upset.

If the child is unable to swallow the tablet, it can be crushed and mixed with water or soft food (such as applesauce, pudding, jam, or jelly). This mixture should be swallowed and not chewed. The entire mixture must be swallowed to ensure that the child received the full dose.

Special Instructions

May cause drowsiness or dizziness in some people. Until it is known how the child will react to the medicine, activities that require mental alertness (such as physical education and playground activity) should be restricted.

May cause dizziness upon standing; therefore, always have the child stand up slowly. If the child becomes dizzy, he should be instructed to sit or lie down immediately.

For older children, dry mouth may be relieved by chewing gum or sucking on hard candy or ice chips. Younger children may need extra liquids.

The child may have to wear sunglasses outside, because this medicine may cause his eyes to become more sensitive to sunlight.

Benztropine mesylate increases the chance of heat stroke because it decreases the child's ability to sweat; therefore, physical education and playground activity should be restricted, especially on hot days.

Notes

B ethanechol chloride

Brand Names

Duvoid
(tablet)
Myotonachol
(tablet)
Urecholine
(tablet)

Common Uses

Bethanechol belongs to the class of medicines called cholinergics. Bethanechol is used to treat conditions in which the child's airway is hurt by stomach acid (gastroesophageal reflux) and treat children who have difficulty urinating. Bethanechol is able to treat these conditions by imitating a chemical that helps treat these problems.

Usual Dose

Children

GASTROESOPHAGEAL REFLUX: 0.1–0.2 mg/kg/dose given 4 times a day.

URINATION DIFFICULTY: 0.6 mg/kg/day divided into equal doses given every 6–8 hours.

Adults: 10–50 mg/dose given every 6–12 hours.

Medication Interactions

Medications that may increase the risk for the development of bethanechol adverse side effects are:

ambenonium

neostigmine

pyridostigmine

Medications that may decrease the effectiveness of bethanechol are:

procainamide

quinidine

A medication that may cause a dangerous decrease in blood pressure when combined with bethanechol is:

mecamylamine

Adverse Side Effects

Minor: Nausea, vomiting, diarrhea, stomach cramps, headache, dizziness, increased salivation, sweating, blurred vision.

Severe: Chest pain, difficulty breathing, wheezing, fainting.

Storage and Administration

The oral medicine should be stored in a cool, dry place away from light. Prolonged exposure to heat, moisture, or light can damage the medicine.

Bethanechol should be taken on an empty stomach (1 hour before a meal or 2–3 hours after a meal). If taken with food, nausea and vomiting can occur.

If the child is unable to swallow the bethanechol tablet, it can be crushed and mixed with a small amount of water. The entire mixture must be swallowed to ensure that the child received the full dose.

Special Instructions

May cause dizziness in some children. Until it is known how the child will react to the medicine, activities that require mental alertness (such as physical education and playground activity) should be restricted.

May cause dizziness upon standing; therefore, always have the child stand up slowly. If the child becomes dizzy, she should be instructed to sit or lie down immediately.

N o t e s

B rompheniramine maleate

Brand Names

Bromphen
(liquid)

Diamine T.D.
(long-acting
tablet)

Dimetane
(tablet, liquid)

Dimetane
Extentabs
(long-acting
tablet)

Veltane
(tablet)

Common Uses

Brompheniramine belongs to the class of medicines called antihistamines. Brompheniramine is used to treat seasonal and constant runny noses due to allergies and colds by blocking the chemical histamine, which causes these problems.

Usual Dose

Children younger than 6 years: 0.125 mg/kg/dose divided into equal doses given every 6 hours. Maximum dose 6–8 mg/day.

Children 6–12 years old: 2–4 mg/dose given every 6–8 hours. Maximum dose 12–16 mg/day.

Children older than 12 years and Adults: 4 mg/dose given every 4–6 hours. If the long-acting medicine is being used, the dose is 8–12 mg/dose every 8–12 hours. Maximum dose 24 mg/day.

Medication Interactions

Medications that may increase the risk of sedation, drowsiness, and dizziness when combined with brompheniramine are:

alcohol	fluphenazine
amitriptyline	nortriptyline
amoxapine	perphenazine
clomipramine	prochlorperazine
desipramine	thioridazine
doxepin	trifluoperazine

Adverse Side Effects

Minor: Drowsiness; dizziness; sedation; dry mouth, nose and throat; nausea; headache; upset stomach; sweating; constipation; increased sensitivity to sunlight.

Severe: Sore throat, fever, unusual bruising or bleeding, rash, clumsiness, hallucinations, fast heartbeat, awareness of heartbeat, seizures, difficulty breathing, chest tightness, fatigue, weakness, blurred vision.

Storage and Administration

The oral medicine should be stored in a cool, dry place away from light. Prolonged exposure to heat, moisture, or light can damage the medicine.

The liquid may be stored at room temperature and does not need to be refrigerated.

If upset stomach occurs, brompheniramine can be given with food.

The tablet and long-acting tablet should be swallowed whole with a full glass of water. Do not crush or allow the child to chew it.

Special Instructions

May cause sedation, drowsiness, and dizziness in some people. Until it is known how the child will react to the medicine, activities that require mental alertness (such as physical education and playground activity) should be restricted.

In children with a seizure disorder, this medicine may cause seizures even if the seizures are currently controlled.

For older children, dry mouth may be relieved by chewing gum or sucking on hard candy or ice chips. Younger children may need extra liquids.

Have the child avoid prolonged exposure to sunlight because this medication may cause him to be more sensitive to it.

N o t e s

C aptopril

Common Uses

Captopril belongs to the class of medicines called angiotensin-converting enzyme inhibitors (ACE inhibitors). Captopril is used to treat and control high blood pressure and weak hearts because it blocks angiotensin-converting enzyme from producing angiotensin II, a chemical that causes blood vessels to narrow.

Usual Dose

Infants: 0.15–0.3 mg/kg/dose given 1–4 times a day. Adjust the dose according to the physician's directions until the desired effect is obtained. Maximum dose 6 mg/kg/day.

Children: 0.5 mg/kg/dose given 1–4 times a day. Adjust the dose according to the physician's directions until the desired effect is obtained. Maximum dose 6 mg/kg/day.

Older Children: 6.25–12.5 mg/dose given 1–2 times a day. Adjust the dose according to the physician's directions until the desired effect is obtained. Maximum dose 6 mg/kg/day.

Adolescents and Adults: 12.5–25 mg/dose given 2–3 times a day. Adjust the dose according to the physician's directions until the desired effect is obtained. Maximum dose 450 mg/day.

Medication Interactions

A medication that may decrease the therapeutic effect of captopril is:

indomethacin

Adverse Side Effects

Minor: Nausea, vomiting, diarrhea, constipation, upset stomach, dizziness, dry mouth, flushing, headache, insomnia, loss of taste, dry cough, increased sensitivity to sunlight.

C

Severe: Chest pain; fever; chills; rash; sore throat or mouth; mouth sores; awareness of heartbeat; abnormal heartbeat; prolonged or persistent nausea, vomiting, or diarrhea; persistent fatigue; continued or intermittent dizziness; swelling of mouth, face, feet, or hands; feeling of heaviness in legs; unusual bruising or bleeding; yellow skin or eyes; tingling or numbness in fingers, toes, or lips; difficulty breathing; unusual fatigue or weakness; unexplained nervousness; fainting; confusion; cloudy urine; darkened nailbeds.

Storage and Administration

The oral medicine should be stored in a cool, dry place away from light. Prolonged exposure to heat, moisture, or light can damage the medicine.

Captopril should be taken on an empty stomach (1 hour before a meal or 2–3 hours after a meal).

If the child is unable to swallow the captopril tablet, it can be crushed and mixed with a small amount of water. This mixture should be swallowed and not chewed. The entire mixture must be swallowed to ensure that the child received the full dose.

Special Instructions

May cause dizziness upon standing; therefore, always have the child stand up slowly. If the child becomes dizzy, she should be instructed to sit or lie down immediately.

The child should avoid prolonged exposure to sunlight—this medication may cause her to be more sensitive to it.

For older children, dry mouth may be relieved by chewing gum or sucking on hard candy or ice chips. Younger children may need extra liquids.

N o t e s

Carbamazepine

Brand Names

Epitol
(tablet)
Tegretol
(chewable
tablet, tablet,
liquid)

Common Uses

Carbamazepine belongs to the class of medicines called anticonvulsants. Carbamazepine is used to treat and control seizures by decreasing the ability of the seizure to spread throughout the brain. Carbamazepine also is used to relieve nerve pain and to treat people with manic-depressive disorder.

Usual Dose

Children younger than 6 years: 5–20 mg/kg/day divided into equal doses given 2–4 times a day.

Children 6-12 years old: 10–30 mg/kg/day divided into equal doses given 2–4 times a day.

Children older than 12 years and Adults: 400–1200 mg/day divided into equal doses given 3–4 times a day.

Medication Interactions

Medications that may increase the risk for the development of carbamazepine adverse side effects are:

azithromycin   fluoxetine

cimetidine   isoniazid

clarithromycin   troleandomycin

diltiazem   valproic acid

divalproex sodium   verapamil

erythromycin

Medications that may decrease the effectiveness of carbamazepine are:

felbamate   phenytoin

phenobarbital   primidone

Carbamazepine increases the risk for the development of adverse side effects of:

isoniazid

phenytoin

Carbamazepine decreases the effectiveness of:

dicumarol	haloperidol
divalproex sodium	phenytoin
doxycycline	valproic acid
felbamate	warfarin

A medication that may cause drowsiness, fatigue, muscle weakness, and tremor when combined with carbamazepine is:

lithium

Adverse Side Effects

Minor: Nausea, diarrhea, constipation, dry mouth, blurred vision, upset stomach, drowsiness, sedation, dizziness, agitation, confusion, headache, muscle or joint pain, increased sensitivity to sunlight.

Severe: Hallucination, hives, rash, sore throat, fever, unusual bruising or bleeding, yellow skin or eyes, stomach pain, difficulty breathing, loss of balance, mouth sores, numbness and tingling in hands or feet, swelling of hands or feet, unusual eye movements.

Storage and Administration

The oral medicine should be stored in a cool, dry place away from light. Prolonged exposure to heat, moisture, or light can damage the medicine.

Before measuring the dose, the liquid form of carbamazepine should be shaken well. The liquid may be stored at room temperature and does not need to be refrigerated.

It is best to take this medicine with food or milk to decrease or prevent stomach upset.

C

The chewable tablet should be chewed thoroughly before swallowing.

If the child is unable to swallow the nonchewable tablet, it can be crushed and mixed with small amount of water or soft food (such as applesauce, pudding, jam, or jelly). This mixture should be swallowed and not chewed. The entire mixture must be swallowed to ensure that the child received the full dose.

Special Instructions

May cause sedation, drowsiness, and dizziness in some people. Until it is known how the child will react to the medicine, activities that require mental alertness (such as physical education and playground activity) should be restricted.

Do not suddenly stop giving carbamazepine to the child unless instructed to do so by a physician. Suddenly stopping this medication may cause severe seizures to occur.

For older children, dry mouth may be relieved by chewing gum or sucking on hard candy or ice chips. Younger children may need extra liquids.

Have the child avoid prolonged exposure to sunlight because this medication may cause him to be more sensitive to it.

N o t e s

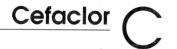

Common Uses

Cefaclor belongs to the class of medicines called antibiotics, which are used to treat a variety of bacterial infections. Cefaclor is prescribed for infections of the middle ear, respiratory tract, urinary tract, skin, bones, and joints, because it prevents the bacteria from growing.

Cefaclor is effective only in the treatment of bacterial infections, not those caused by viruses, parasites, or yeast.

Usual Dose

Children older than 1 month: 20–40 mg/kg/day divided into equal doses given every 8–12 hours. Maximum dose 2 g/day.

Adults: 250–500 mg/dose given every 8 hours.

Medication Interactions

No major medication interactions have been found with other oral medications.

Adverse Side Effects

Minor: Nausea, vomiting, diarrhea, dizziness, upset stomach, headache.

Severe: Rash, hives, difficulty breathing, seizures, severe diarrhea, unusual bruising or bleeding, stomach cramps, fatigue, joint pain, fever.

Storage and Administration

The oral medicine should be stored in a cool, dry place away from light. Prolonged exposure to heat, moisture, or light can damage the medicine.

Before the dose is measured, the liquid form of cefaclor should be shaken well. Refrigeration of the liquid is recommended. After receiving the liquid medicine from the pharmacy, it is good only for 14 days; therefore, always check the expiration date on the prescription label before using.

Brand Name
Ceclor (capsule, liquid)

If upset stomach occurs, cefaclor can be given with food or milk.

If the child is unable to swallow the capsule, it can be opened and mixed with soft food (such as applesauce, pudding, jam, or jelly). This mixture should be swallowed and not chewed. The entire mixture must be swallowed to ensure that the child received the full dose.

Special Instructions

The child's physician should be notified if the infection worsens or does not improve within 3–5 days.

May cause dizziness in some people. Until it is known how the child will react to the medicine, activities that require mental alertness (such as physical education and playground activity) should be restricted.

N o t e s

Cefadroxil C

Common Uses

Cefadroxil belongs to the class of medicines called antibiotics, which are used to treat a variety of bacterial infections. Cefadroxil is prescribed for infections of the middle ear, respiratory tract, urinary tract, or other infections, because it prevents the bacteria from growing.

Cefadroxil is effective only against bacterial infections, not those caused by viruses, parasites, or yeast.

Usual Dose

Children: 30 mg/kg/day divided into equal doses given 1–2 times a day. Maximum dose 2 g/day.

Adults: 1–2 g/day divided into equal doses given 1–2 times a day.

Medication Interactions

No major medication interactions have been found with other oral medications.

Adverse Side Effects

Minor: Nausea, vomiting, diarrhea, dizziness, upset stomach, headache.

Severe: Rash, hives, difficulty breathing, seizures, severe diarrhea, unusual bruising or bleeding, stomach cramps, fatigue, joint pain, fever.

Storage and Administration

The oral medicine should be stored in a cool, dry place away from light. Prolonged exposure to heat, moisture, or light can damage the medicine.

Before the dose is measured, the liquid form of cefadroxil should be shaken well. Refrigeration of the liquid is recommended. After receiving the liquid medicine from the pharmacy, it is good only for 14 days; therefore, always check the expiration date on the prescription label before using.

Brand Names

Duricef
(tablet, cap-
sule, liquid)
Ultracef
(tablet, cap-
sule, liquid)

If upset stomach occurs, cefadroxil can be given with food or milk.

If the child is unable to swallow pills, the capsule can be opened or the tablet crushed and mixed with soft food (such as applesauce, pudding, jam, or jelly). This mixture should be swallowed and not chewed. The entire mixture must be swallowed to ensure that the child received the full dose.

Special Instructions

Notify the child's physician if the infection worsens or does not improve within 3–5 days.

May cause dizziness in some people. Until it is known how the child will react to the medicine, activities that require mental alertness (such as physical education and playground activity) should be restricted.

N o t e s

Cefixime C

Common Uses

Cefixime belongs to the class of medicines called antibiotics, which are used to treat a variety of bacterial infections. Cefixime is prescribed for infections of the middle ear, respiratory tract, soft tissue, and bone, because it prevents the bacteria from growing.

Cefixime is effective only in the treatment of bacterial infections, not those caused by viruses, parasites, or yeast.

Usual Dose

Children: 8 mg/kg/day divided into equal doses given every 12–24 hours. Maximum dose 400 mg/day.

Children older than 12 years, Children weighing more than 50 kg (110 lb), and Adults: 400 mg/day given every 12–24 hours.

Medication Interactions

No major medication interactions have been found with other oral medication.

Adverse Side Effects

Minor: Nausea, vomiting, diarrhea, dizziness, upset stomach, headache.

Severe: Rash, hives, difficulty breathing, seizures, severe diarrhea, unusual bruising or bleeding, stomach cramps, fatigue, joint pain, fever.

Storage and Administration

The oral medicine should be stored in a cool, dry place away from light. Prolonged exposure to heat, moisture, or light can damage the medicine.

Before the dose is measured, the liquid form of cefixime should be shaken well. The liquid may be stored at room temperature and does not need to be refrigerated. After receiving the liquid medicine from the pharmacy, it is good only for 14 days; therefore, always check the expiration date on the prescription label before using.

Brand Name

Suprax
(tablet, liquid)

C

If upset stomach occurs, the medicine can be given with food or milk.

If the child is unable to swallow the tablet, it can be crushed and mixed with soft food (such as applesauce, pudding, jam, or jelly). This mixture should be swallowed and not chewed. The entire mixture must be swallowed to ensure that the child received the full dose.

Special Instructions

The child's physician should be notified if the infection worsens or does not improve within 3–5 days.

May cause dizziness in some people. Until it is known how the child will react to the medicine, activities that require mental alertness (such as physical education and playground activity) should be restricted.

Notes

Cefpodoxime proxetil

Common Uses

Cefpodoxime belongs to the class of medicines called antibiotics, which are used to treat a variety of bacterial infections. Cefpodoxime is prescribed for infections of the middle ear, respiratory tract, urinary tract, and skin, because it prevents the bacteria from growing.

Cefpodoxime is effective only against bacterial infections, not those caused by viruses, parasites, or yeast.

Usual Dose

Children 6 months–12 years old: 5 mg/kg/dose given every 12 hours.

Children older than 12 years and Adults: 100–400 mg/dose given every 12 hours.

Medication Interactions

No major medication interactions have been found with other oral medications.

Adverse Side Effects

Minor: Nausea, vomiting, diarrhea, dizziness, upset stomach, headache.

Severe: Rash, hives, difficulty breathing, seizures, severe diarrhea, unusual bruising or bleeding, stomach cramps, fatigue, joint pain, fever.

Storage and Administration

The oral medicine should be stored in a cool, dry place away from light. Prolonged exposure to heat, moisture, or light can damage the medicine.

Before the dose is measured, the liquid form of cefpodoxime should be shaken well. Refrigeration of the liquid is recommended. After receiving the liquid medicine from the pharmacy, it is good only for 14 days; therefore, always check the expiration date on the prescription label before using.

This medicine should be given with food to increase the amount that the body absorbs.

Brand Name
Vantin (tablet, liquid)

If the child is unable to swallow the tablet, it can be crushed and mixed with soft food (such as applesauce, pudding, jam, or jelly). This mixture should be swallowed and not chewed. The entire mixture must be swallowed to ensure that the child received the full dose.

Special Instructions

The child's physician should be notified if the infection worsens or does not improve within 3–5 days.

May cause dizziness in some people. Until it is known how the child will react to the medicine, activities that require mental alertness (such as physical education and playground activity) should be restricted.

N o t e s

Cefprozil C

Common Uses

Cefprozil belongs to the class of medicines called antibiotics, which are used to treat a variety of bacterial infections. Cefprozil is prescribed for infections of the middle ear and skin, because it prevents the bacteria from growing.

Cefprozil is effective only against bacterial infections, not those caused by viruses, parasites, or yeast.

Usual Dose

Children 6 months–12 years old: 7.5–15 mg/kg/dose given twice a day.

Children older than 12 years and Adults: 250–500 mg/dose given 1–2 times a day.

Medication Interactions

No major medication interactions have been found with other oral medications.

Adverse Side Effects

Minor: Nausea, vomiting, diarrhea, dizziness, upset stomach, headache.

Severe: Rash, hives, difficulty breathing, seizures, severe diarrhea, unusual bruising or bleeding, stomach cramps, fatigue, joint pain, fever.

Storage and Administration

The oral medicine should be stored in a cool, dry place away from light. Prolonged exposure to heat, moisture, or light can damage the medicine.

Before the dose is measured, the liquid form of cefprozil should be shaken well. Refrigeration of the liquid is recommended. After receiving the liquid medicine from the pharmacy, it is good only for 14 days; therefore, always check the expiration date on the prescription label before using.

If upset stomach occurs, the medicine can be given with food or milk.

Brand Name

Cefzil
(tablet, liquid)

If the child is unable to swallow the tablet, it can be crushed and mixed with soft food (such as applesauce, pudding, jam, or jelly). This mixture should be swallowed and not chewed. The entire mixture must be swallowed to ensure that the child received the full dose.

Special Instructions

The child's physician should be notified if the infection worsens or does not improve within 3–5 days.

May cause dizziness in some people. Until it is known how the child will react to the medicine, activities that require mental alertness (such as physical education and playground activity) should be restricted.

N o t e s

Cefuroxime axetil C

Common Uses

Cefuroxime axetil belongs to the class of medicines called antibiotics, which are used to treat a variety of bacterial infections. Cefuroxime axetil is prescribed for infections of the middle ear, respiratory tract, urinary tract, skin, soft tissue, bones, and joints, because it prevents the bacteria from growing.

Cefuroxime axetil is effective only against bacterial infections, not those caused by viruses, parasites, or yeast.

Usual Dose

TABLET

Children 2–12 years old: 125–250 mg/dose given twice a day.

Children older than 12 years and Adults: 125–500 mg/dose given twice a day.

LIQUID

Children 3 months–12 years old: 20–30 mg/kg/day divided into equal doses given twice a day. Maximum dose 1000 mg/day.

Medication Interactions

No major medication interactions have been found with other oral medications.

Adverse Side Effects

Minor: Nausea, vomiting, diarrhea, dizziness, upset stomach, headache.

Severe: Rash, hives, difficulty breathing, seizures, severe diarrhea, unusual bruising or bleeding, stomach cramps, fatigue, joint pain, fever.

Storage and Administration

The oral medicine should be stored in a cool, dry place away from light. Prolonged exposure to heat, moisture, or light can damage the medicine.

Brand Name
Ceftin **(tablet, liquid)**

It is best not to crush the tablets because the powder has a very bitter taste.

The liquid should be shaken well. The medicine may be kept in the refrigerator or at room temperature. Any unused portion should be discarded after 10 days.

Cefuroxime axetil should be taken with food or milk.

Special Instructions

The child's physician should be notified if the infection worsens or does not improve within 3–5 days.

May cause dizziness in some people. Until it is known how the child will react to the medicine, activities that require mental alertness (such as physical education and playground activity) should be restricted.

Notes

Cephalexin C

Common Uses

Cephalexin belongs to the class of medicines called antibiotics, which are used to treat a variety of bacterial infections. Cephalexin is prescribed for infections of the middle ear, respiratory tract, and urinary tract, because it prevents the bacteria from growing.

Cephalexin is effective only against bacterial infections, not those caused by viruses, parasites, or yeast.

Usual Dose

Children: 25–100 mg/kg/day divided into equal doses given every 6 hours. Maximum dose 4 g/day.

Adults: 250–500 mg/dose every 6 hours. In some situations the medicine may be given every 12 hours.

Medication Interactions

No major medication interactions have been found with other oral medications.

Adverse Side Effects

Minor: Nausea, vomiting, diarrhea, dizziness, upset stomach, headache.

Severe: Rash, hives, difficulty breathing, seizures, severe diarrhea, unusual bruising or bleeding, stomach cramps, fatigue, joint pain, fever.

Storage and Administration

The oral medicine should be stored in a cool, dry place away from light. Prolonged exposure to heat, moisture, or light can damage the medicine.

Before measuring the dose, the liquid form of cephalexin should be shaken well. Refrigeration of the liquid is recommended. After receiving the liquid medicine from the pharmacy, it is good only for 14 days; therefore, always check the expiration date on the prescription label before using.

Brand Name

Keflet
  (tablet)
Keflex
  (capsule,
  liquid)
Keftab
  (tablet)

If upset stomach occurs, cephalexin can be given with food or milk.

If the child is unable to swallow pills, the tablets can be crushed or the capsules opened and mixed with water or soft food (such as applesauce, pudding, jam, or jelly). This mixture should be swallowed and not chewed. The entire mixture must be swallowed to ensure that the child received the full dose.

Special Instructions

The child's physician should be notified if the infection worsens or does not improve within 3–5 days.

May cause dizziness in some people. Until it is known how the child will react to the medicine, activities that require mental alertness (such as physical education and playground activity) should be restricted.

N o t e s

Cephradine C

Common Uses

Cephradine belongs to the class of medicines called antibiotics, which are used to treat a variety of bacterial infections. Cephradine is prescribed for infections of the middle ear, respiratory tract, and urinary tract, because it prevents the bacteria from growing.

Cephradine treats only bacterial infections, not those caused by viruses, parasites, or yeast.

Usual Dose

Children older than 9 months: 25–100 mg/kg/day divided into equal doses given every 6–12 hours. Maximum dose 4 g/day.

Adults: 250–500 mg/dose given every 6 hours or 500–1000 mg given every 12 hours. Maximum dose 4 g/day.

Medication Interactions

No major medication interactions have been found with other oral medications.

Adverse Side Effects

Minor: Nausea, vomiting, diarrhea, dizziness, upset stomach, headache.

Severe: Rash, hives, difficulty breathing, seizures, severe diarrhea, unusual bruising or bleeding, stomach cramps, fatigue, joint pain, fever.

Storage and Administration

The oral medicine should be stored in a cool, dry place away from light. Prolonged exposure to heat, moisture, or light can damage the medicine.

Before the dose is measured, the liquid form of cephradine should be shaken well. Refrigeration of the liquid is recommended. After receiving the liquid medicine from the pharmacy, it is good only for 14

Brand Name
Velosef (capsule, liquid)

days; therefore, always check the expiration date on the prescription label before using.

If upset stomach occurs, the medicine can be given with food.

If the child is unable to swallow the capsule, it can be opened and mixed with soft food (such as applesauce, pudding, jam, or jelly). This mixture should be swallowed and not chewed. The entire mixture must be swallowed to ensure that the child received the full dose.

Special Instructions

The child's physician should be notified if the infection worsens or does not improve within 3–5 days.

May cause dizziness in some people. Until it is known how the child will react to the medicine, activities that require mental alertness (such as physical education and playground activity) should be restricted.

N o t e s

Chlorpheniramine maleate

Common Uses

Chlorpheniramine maleate belongs to the class of medicines called antihistamines. Chlorphen-iramine is used to treat sneezing and runny noses caused by allergies and colds, because it blocks the chemical histamine, which causes these problems.

Usual Dose

Children 2–6 years old: 1 mg/dose given every 4–6 hours. Maximum dose 4 mg/day.

Children 6–12 years old: 2 mg/dose given every 4–6 hours. The usual dose of the long-acting tablet is 8 mg/dose once a day. Maximum dose 12 mg/day.

Children older than 12 years and Adults: 4 mg/dose given every 4–6 hours. The usual dose of the long-acting tablet is 8–12 mg/dose given every 8–12 hours. Maximum dose 24 mg/day.

Medication Interactions

Medications that may increase the risk of sedation, drowsiness, and dizziness when combined with chlorpheniramine are:

alcohol	fluphenazine
amitriptyline	nortriptyline
amoxapine	perphenazine
clomipramine	prochlorperazine
desipramine	thioridazine
doxepin	trifluoperazine

Brand Names

Aller-Chlor
(tablet, liquid)

Chlo-Amine
(chewable
tablet)

Chlorate
(tablet)

Chlortab-4
(tablet)

Chlortab-8
(long-acting
tablet)

Chlor-Trimeton
(tablet, liquid)

Chlor-Trimeton
Repetabs
(long-acting
tablet)

Phenetron
(tablet, liquid)

Telachlor
(long-acting
capsule)

Adverse Side Effects

Minor: Drowsiness; dizziness; sedation; dry mouth, nose, or throat; nausea; headache; upset stomach; sweating; constipation; increased sensitivity to sunlight.

Severe: Sore throat, fever, unusual bruising or bleeding, rash, clumsiness, hallucinations, fast heartbeat, awareness of heartbeat, seizures, difficulty breathing, chest tightness, weakness, fatigue, blurred vision.

Storage and Administration

The oral medicine should be stored in a cool, dry place away from light. Prolonged exposure to heat, moisture, or light can damage the medicine.

The liquid may be stored at room temperature and does not need to be refrigerated.

If upset stomach occurs, chlorpheniramine can be given with food.

The chewable tablet should be chewed thoroughly before swallowing.

The long-acting tablet and long-acting capsule should be swallowed whole with a full glass of water. Do not crush or allow the child to chew them.

If the child is unable to swallow the non–long-acting tablet, it can be crushed and mixed with soft food (such as applesauce, pudding, jam, or jelly). This mixture should be swallowed and not chewed. The entire mixture must be swallowed to ensure that the child received the full dose.

Special Instructions

May cause sedation, drowsiness, and dizziness in some people. Until it is known how the child will react to the medicine, activities that require mental alertness (such as physical education and playground activity) should be restricted.

May cause dizziness upon standing; therefore, always have the child stand up slowly. If the child becomes dizzy he should be instructed to sit or lie down immediately.

In children with a seizure disorder, this medicine may cause seizures even if the seizures are currently controlled.

For older children, dry mouth may be relieved by chewing gum or sucking on hard candy or ice chips. Younger children may need extra liquids.

The child should avoid prolonged exposure to sunlight, because this medication may cause him to be more sensitive to it.

Notes

C hlorpromazine hydrochloride

Brand Names

Thorazine
(tablet, liquid,
concentrate,
rectal
suppository)

Thorazine
Spansules
(long-acting
capsules)

Common Uses

Chlorpromazine belongs to the class of medicines called tranquilizers. Chlorpromazine is used to treat various forms of mental illness and agitation because it blocks chemicals responsible for imbalanced nerve transmission in the brain.

Usual Dose

MENTAL ILLNESS AND AGITATION

Children older than 6 months: 0.5–1 mg/kg/dose given every 4–6 hours.

Adults: Start with 30 mg/day divided into equal doses given 1–4 times a day. Increase the dose as directed by the physician until the desired effect occurs. Maximum dose 2000 mg/day.

NAUSEA AND VOMITING

ORAL

Children older than 6 months: 0.5–1 mg/kg/dose given every 4–6 hours as needed.

Adults: 10–25 mg/dose given every 4–6 hours as needed.

RECTAL SUPPOSITORY

See the Medication Administration section for instructions on the proper use of a rectal suppository (page 18).

Children older than 6 months: 1 mg/kg/dose given every 6–8 hours as needed.

Adults: 50–100 mg/dose given every 6–8 hours as needed.

Medication Interactions

Medications that may increase the risk for the development of chlorpromazine adverse side effects are:

alcohol

meperidine

propranolol

Medications that may decrease the effectiveness of chlorpromazine are:

atropine   scopolamine

benztropine   trihexyphenidyl

oxybutynin

Chlorpromazine may decrease the effectiveness of:

guanethidine

propranolol

Adverse Side Effects

Minor: Vomiting, diarrhea, constipation, dizziness, drowsiness, stuffy nose, dry mouth, restlessness, discolored urine, increased sensitivity to sunlight, blurred vision, weight gain.

Severe: Chest pain; seizures; difficulty swallowing or breathing; fever; sore throat; rash; stomach pain; yellow skin or eyes; unusual bruising or bleeding; trembling; twitching; drooling; unintentional movements of face, mouth, and tongue.

Storage and Administration

The oral medicine should be stored in a cool, dry place away from light. Prolonged exposure to heat, moisture, or light can damage the medicine.

The liquid and concentrate may be stored at room temperature and do not need to be refrigerated.

The rectal suppositories may be stored at room temperature and do not need to be refrigerated.

Keep the concentrate out of sunlight because this will damage the medicine.

Chlorpromazine works best if taken on an empty stomach (1 hour before a meal or 2–3 hours after a meal). However, if upset stomach occurs, it can be given with food or milk.

The long-acting capsule should be swallowed whole with a full glass of water. Do not crush or allow the child to chew it.

If the child is unable to swallow the tablet, it can be crushed and mixed with soft food (such as applesauce, pudding, jam, or jelly). This mixture should be swallowed and not chewed. The entire mixture must be swallowed to ensure that the child received the full dose.

Do not touch the regular liquid form or concentrate, or allow it to touch the child's skin because it may produce an itchy rash.

The concentrate must be mixed with half a cup or more of orange juice, milk, or water, or with a small amount of soft food (such as applesauce, pudding, jam, or jelly). The child must drink or eat all of the mixture. Prepare the mixture just before giving the dose. The medicine will be damaged if left in the mixture; therefore, do not premix and store.

Special Instructions

May cause sedation, drowsiness, and dizziness in some people. Until it is known how the child will react to the medicine, activities that require mental alertness (such as physical education and playground activity) should be restricted.

May cause dizziness upon standing; therefore, always have the child stand up slowly. If the child becomes dizzy, she should be instructed to sit or lie down immediately.

Limit playing on hot days because the medicine increases the risk of heat stroke.

For older children, dry mouth may be relieved by chewing gum or sucking on hard candy or ice chips. Younger children may need extra liquids.

In children with a seizure disorder, this medicine may cause seizures even
if the child's condition is currently controlled.

May cause the urine to become pink, purple, or red-brown in color. This occurs frequently and is harmless.

Have the child avoid prolonged exposure to sunlight because chlorpheniramine may cause him to be more sensitive to it.

If the child suddenly stops taking chlorpromazine, nausea, vomiting, upset stomach, headache, fast heartbeat, and tremors may develop.

Cimetidine C

Common Uses

Cimetidine belongs to the class of medicines called histamine$_2$-antagonists, which are used to treat and prevent certain types of stomach and upper intestine ulcers. Cimetidine also is used in diseases where there is too much acid in the stomach (hypersecretory conditions) and when the airway is being damaged by stomach acid (gastroesophageal reflux). Cimetidine is able to treat these problems by reducing the amount of acid in the stomach. It blocks histamine, which is responsible for the secretion of acid into the stomach.

Usual Dose

Infants: 10–20 mg/kg/day divided into equal doses given every 6–12 hours.

Children: 20–40 mg/kg/day divided into equal doses given every 6 hours.

Adults

ULCER PREVENTION: 400 mg/dose given at bedtime.

ULCER TREATMENT: 300 mg/dose every 6 hours, 400 mg/dose every 12 hours, or 800 mg once a day at bedtime.

GASTROESOPHAGEAL REFLUX DISEASE: 800 mg/dose every 12 hours or 400 mg/dose every 6 hours.

HYPERSECRETORY CONDITIONS: 300–600 mg/dose every 6 hours. Maximum dose 2400 mg/day. Doses sometimes are given more often.

Medication Interactions

Medications that may decrease the effectiveness of cimetidine are:

antacids

Brand Name
Tagamet (tablet, liquid)

C

Cimetidine increases the risk for the development of adverse side effects of:

amitriptyline	nortriptyline
carbamazepine	phenytoin
clomipramine	procainamide
desipramine	propranolol
doxepin	quinidine
felodipine	rimantadine
imipramine	theophylline
nifedipine	warfarin

Cimetidine decreases the effectiveness of:

ketoconazole

A medication that may cause drowsiness, sedation, and lack of coordination when combined with cimetidine is:

alcohol

Adverse Side Effects

Minor: Dizziness, drowsiness, headache, muscle pain, diarrhea, hair loss, constipation.

Severe: Confusion, fever, hallucinations, rash, sore throat, fever, unusual bruising or bleeding, weakness, yellow skin or eyes, awareness of heartbeat, slow or fast heartbeat, muscle pain, fatigue.

Storage and Administration

The oral medicine should be stored in a cool, dry place away from light. Prolonged exposure to heat, moisture, or light can damage the medicine.

The liquid may be stored at room temperature and does not need to be refrigerated.

It is best to take cimetidine with or shortly after meals and at bedtime to obtain maximum effect.

Do not allow the child to take antacids within 1 hour before or 1 hour after taking cimetidine.

The tablets should be swallowed whole, because cimetidine has a bitter taste and bad odor when crushed or chewed.

Special Instructions

May cause drowsiness and dizziness in some people. Until it is known how the child will react to the medicine, activities that require mental alertness (such as physical education and playground activity) should be restricted.

The child's physician should be notified as soon as possible if vomiting that looks like coffee grounds or has blood in it, or black or bloody stools occur.

N o t e s

C iprofloxacin

Brand Name

Cipro
(tablet)
Ciloxan
(eye drops)

Common Uses

Ciprofloxacin belongs to the class of medicines called antibiotics, which are used to treat a variety of bacterial infections. Oral tablets are prescribed for infections of the respiratory tract, skin, bones, joints, and urinary tract. Eye drops are used to treat bacterial infections of the eyes.

Ciprofloxacin is effective only against bacterial infections, not those caused by viruses, parasites, or yeast.

Usual Dose

TABLETS

Children: 20–30 mg/kg/day divided into equal doses given every 12 hours. Maximum dose 1.5 g/day.

Adults: 250–750 mg/dose given every 12 hours.

Children and Adults with cystic fibrosis have received 40 mg/kg/day divided into equal doses given every 8 hours.

EYE DROPS

See the Medication Administration section for instructions on the proper technique to instill eye drops (page 8).

Children 12 years or older and Adults: 1 drop in each eye every 2 hours while awake for 2 days, then 1 drop in each eye every 4 hours while awake for five days.

Medication Interactions

Medications that may decrease the effectiveness of ciprofloxacin (tablets) are:

antacids   iron supplements

didanosine   sucralfate

Ciprofloxacin (tablets) may increase the risk for the development of adverse side effects of:

theophylline

Adverse Side Effects

Minor: Diarrhea, nausea, upset stomach, headache, dizziness, insomnia, increased sensitivity to sunlight.

Severe: Blood in the urine, seizures, confusion, persistent dizziness, hallucinations, lower back or joint pain, painful or difficult urination, rash, trembling, bad taste in the mouth, unusual bruising or bleeding, yellow skin or eyes, ringing in the ears, eye pain, blurred or double vision, dry mouth, vomiting.

Storage and Administration

The oral medicine should be stored in a cool, dry place away from light. Prolonged exposure to heat, moisture, or light can damage the medicine.

Do not allow the child to take antacids within 4 hours before or 2 hours after taking ciprofloxacin.

Do not allow the child to take sucralfate 2 hours before or 2 hours after taking ciprofloxacin.

Ciprofloxacin should be taken with a full glass of water and at least 3 full glasses of water between doses.

Ciprofloxacin works best if taken 2 hours after a meal, but if upset stomach occurs, it can be given with food.

It is best not to crush the tablets due to the bad taste of the powder. However, if necessary, the tablets can be crushed and mixed with a small amount of water or soft food (such as applesauce, pudding, jam, or jelly). This mixture should be swallowed and not chewed. The entire mixture must be swallowed to ensure that the child received the full dose.

Special Instructions

The child's physician should be notified if the infection worsens or does not improve within 3–5 days.

May cause dizziness in some people. Until it is known how the child will react to the medicine, activities that require mental alertness (such as physical education and playground activity) should be restricted.

Do not allow the child to drink products with caffeine or eat excessive amounts of chocolate, because caffeine-related side effects (trembling, nervousness, insomnia, fast heartbeat) are more likely to occur.

Have the child avoid prolonged exposure to sunlight because this medication may cause him to be more sensitive to it.

C larithromycin

Brand Name

Biaxin
(film-coated
tablet, liquid)

Common Uses

Clarithromycin belongs to the class of medicines called antibiotics, which are used to treat a variety of bacterial infections. Clarithromycin is prescribed for infections of the respiratory tract and skin, because it prevents the bacteria from growing.

Clarithromycin is effective only against bacterial infections, not those caused by viruses, parasites, or yeast.

Usual Dose

Children: 15 mg/kg/day divided into equal doses given every 12 hours.

Adults: 250–500 mg/dose given every 12 hours.

Medication Interactions

Clarithromycin may increase the risk for the development of adverse side effects of:

astemizole   terfenadine

carbamazepine   theophylline

loratadine

Adverse Side Effects

Minor: Nausea, diarrhea, upset stomach, indigestion, headache, change in taste.

Severe: Persistent diarrhea, fever, loss of hearing, rash, yellow skin or eyes.

Storage and Administration

The oral medicine should be stored in a cool, dry place away from light. Prolonged exposure to heat, moisture, or light can damage the medicine.

Before the dose is measured, the liquid form of clarithromycin should be shaken well. The liquid may be stored at room temperature and does not need to be refrigerated. After receiving the liquid medicine from the pharmacy, it is good only for 14 days; therefore, always check the expiration date on the prescription label before using.

If upset stomach occurs, clarithromycin can be given with food.

The film-coated tablet should be swallowed whole with a full glass of water. Do not crush or allow the child to chew it.

Special Instructions

The child's physician should be notified if the infection worsens or does not improve within 3–5 days.

N o t e s

C lindamycin hydrochloride

Brand Names

Cleocin
(capsule,
liquid)
Cleocin T
(skin gel, skin
solution)

Common Uses

Clindamycin belongs to the class of medicines called antibiotics, which are used to treat a variety of bacterial infections. Clindamycin is prescribed for infections of the respiratory tract, skin, and soft tissue, because it prevents the bacteria from growing. When applied to the skin, clindamycin can be used to treat severe acne.

Clindamycin is effective only against bacterial infections, not those caused by viruses, parasites, or yeast.

Usual Dose

CAPSULE AND LIQUID

Children: 10–30 mg/kg/day divided into equal doses given every 6–8 hours.

Adults: 150–450 mg/dose given every 6–8 hours. Maximum dose 1.8 g/day.

SKIN GEL AND SOLUTION

Children and Adults: Apply as instructed to the infected areas 2 times a day.

Medication Interactions

Medications that may decrease the effectiveness of clindamycin (capsules and liquid) are:

  antacids

Adverse Side Effects

Minor

CAPSULE AND LIQUID: Nausea, upset stomach, loss of appetite, diarrhea, stomach and throat irritation.

SKIN MEDICINE: Dry or oily skin, mild burning or stinging sensation, itching, minor rash, diarrhea, headache, nausea.

Severe: Hives, rash, skin blistering, severe or persistent skin irritation, wheezing, itching, stomach cramps, joint pain, fatigue, weakness, severe diarrhea, blood or pus in the diarrhea, unusual bruising or bleeding, yellow skin or eyes.

Storage and Administration

The oral medicine should be stored in a cool, dry place away from light. Prolonged exposure to heat, moisture, or light can damage the medicine.

Before the dose is measured, the liquid form of clindamycin should be shaken well. The liquid may be stored at room temperature and does not need to be refrigerated. After receiving the liquid medicine from the pharmacy, it is good only for 14 days; therefore, always check the expiration date on the prescription label before using.

The skin gel and solution may be stored at room temperature.

Capsules should be taken with a full glass of water or with food to prevent throat irritation.

If the child is unable to swallow the capsule, it can be opened and mixed with soft food (such as applesauce, pudding, jam, or jelly). This mixture should be swallowed and not chewed. The entire mixture must be swallowed to ensure that the child received the full dose.

If upset stomach occurs, clindamycin can be given with food.

Do not allow the child to take antacids within 2 hours before or 2 hours after taking clindamycin.

Special Instructions

The child's physician should be notified if the infection worsens or does not improve within 3–5 days.

Skin gel and solution are to be used only on the skin; be careful not to get it into the child's eyes.

Report to the child's physician any continuous or severe diarrhea.

N o t e s

C lonazepam

Brand Name

Klonopin
(tablet)

Common Uses

Clonazepam belongs to the class of medicines called anticonvulsants. Clonazepam is used to treat and control seizures by decreasing the ability of the seizure to spread throughout the brain.

Usual Dose

Children younger than 10 years or who weigh less than 30 kg (66 lb): 0.01–0.03 mg/kg/day divided into equal doses given 2–3 times a day. Increase the dose as directed by the physician until the desired effect is achieved. Maximum dose 0.2 mg/kg/day.

Children older than 10 years and Adults: Start with 1.5 mg/day divided into equal doses given 3 times a day. Increase the dose as directed by the physician until the desired effect is achieved. Maximum dose 20 mg/day.

Medication Interactions

A medication that may increase the risk for the development of clonazepam adverse side effects is:

alcohol

Adverse Side Effects

Minor: Drowsiness, sedation, headache, diarrhea, nausea, dry mouth, constipation, insomnia.

Severe: Confusion, depression, fever, hallucinations, muscle weakness, rash, sore gums, trembling, unusual bruising or bleeding, awareness of heartbeat, unusual eye movements.

Storage and Administration:

The oral medicine should be stored in a cool, dry place away from light. Prolonged exposure to heat, moisture, or light can damage the medicine.

If upset stomach occurs, the medicine can be given with food or milk.

If the child is unable to swallow the clonazepam tablet, it can be crushed and mixed with a small amount of water or soft food (such as applesauce, pudding, jam, or jelly). This mixture should be swallowed and not chewed. The entire mixture must be swallowed to ensure that the child received the full dose.

Special Instructions

May cause sedation and drowsiness in some people. Until it is known how the child will react to clonazepam, activities that require mental alertness (such as physical education and playground activity) should be restricted.

Do not allow the child to suddenly stop taking clonazepam unless instructed to do so by a physician. Suddenly stopping this medicine may cause severe seizures to occur.

N o t e s

C lotrimazole

Brand Names

Lotrimin
 (skin cream,
 skin solution,
 skin lotion)

Lotrimin AF
 (skin cream,
 skin solution)

Mycelex
 (lozenge,
 skin cream,
 skin solution)

Common Uses

Clotrimazole belongs to the class of medicines called antifungals, which are used to treat infections caused by yeast (fungus). Clotrimazole is prescribed for infections of the mouth and skin, because it prevents the yeast from growing.

Antifungals are effective only against yeast infections, not those caused by bacteria, viruses, or parasites.

Usual Dose

LOZENGE

Children older than 3 years and Adults: Dissolve 1 lozenge (10 mg) slowly in the mouth 5 times a day.

SKIN CREAM, SOLUTION, AND LOTION

Children and Adults: Apply as directed to the infected area 2 times a day.

Medication Interactions

No major medication interactions have been found with other oral medications.

Adverse Side Effects

Minor

LOZENGE: Nausea, vomiting, upset stomach, diarrhea, mouth irritation.

SKIN MEDICINE: Dry skin, mild burning or stinging sensation, itching, minor rash.

Severe: Rash; hives; blistering, peeling, or swelling of the skin; yellow skin or eyes; dark-colored urine; unusual fatigue or weakness; stomach pain.

Storage and Administration

The lozenges should be stored in a cool, dry place away from light. Prolonged exposure to heat, moisture, or light can damage the medicine.

The skin cream, solution, and lotion may be stored at room temperature.

The lozenge must be dissolved slowly in the mouth. Do not allow the child to swallow or chew it.

If clotrimazole causes an upset stomach, give the child some food or milk before she takes it.

Special Instructions

The child's physician should be notified if the infection worsens or does not improve within 1 week.

Skin cream, solution, and lotion are to be used only on the skin; be careful not to get it into the child's eyes.

N o t e s

C loxacillin sodium

Brand Names

Cloxapen
(capsule)
Tegopen
(capsule,
liquid)

Common Uses

Cloxacillin belongs to the class of medicines called antibiotics, which are used to treat a variety of bacterial infections. Cloxacillin is prescribed for infections of the respiratory tract, skin, bones, and joints, because it prevents the bacteria from growing.

Cloxacillin is effective only against bacterial infections, not those caused by viruses, parasites, or yeast.

Usual Dose

Children older than 1 month: 50–100 mg/kg/day divided into equal doses given every 6 hours. Maximum dose 4 g/day.

Children who weigh more than 20 kg (44 lb) and Adults: 250–500 mg/dose given every 6 hours.

Medication Interactions

Medications that decrease the effectiveness of cloxacillin are:

demeclocycline	minocycline
doxycycline	oxytetracycline
methacycline	tetracycline

Adverse Side Effects

Minor: Diarrhea, nausea, vomiting, heartburn, upset stomach, darkened tongue.

Severe: Rash, hives, difficulty breathing, blood in the urine, sore throat, fever, stomach cramps, seizures, unexplained bleeding or bruising, severe diarrhea.

Storage and Administration

The oral medicine should be stored in a cool, dry place away from light. Prolonged exposure to heat, moisture, or light can damage the medicine.

Before the dose is measured, the liquid form of cloxacillin should be shaken well. Refrigeration of the liquid is recommended. After receiving the liquid medicine from the pharmacy, it is good only for 14 days; therefore, always check the expiration date on the prescription label before using.

Should be taken on an empty stomach (1 hour before a meal or 2–3 hours after a meal).

If the child is unable to swallow the capsule, it can be opened and mixed with small amount of water. This mixture should be swallowed and not chewed. The entire mixture must be swallowed to ensure that the child received the full dose.

Do not allow the child to drink fruit juice or carbonated beverages 1 hour before or 1 hour after taking cloxacillin.

Special Instructions

The child's physician should be notified if the infection worsens or does not improve within 3–5 days.

N o t e s

Codeine

Brand Name

None

Generic
medicine
dosage form:
Codeine
(tablet,
liquid)

Common Uses

Codeine belongs to both the narcotic analgesic and antitussive medicine classes. Codeine is used to treat mild-to-moderate pain, because it binds to chemical receptors that relieve pain. Codeine also can be used to relieve coughing because it suppresses the urge to cough.

Usual Dose

PAIN RELIEVER

Children: 0.5–1 mg/kg/dose given every 4–6 hours as needed for pain. Maximum dose 60 mg/dose.

Adults: 15–60 mg/dose given every 4–6 hours as needed for pain. Maximum dose 360 mg/day.

COUGH SUPPRESSANT

Children: 1–1.5 mg/kg/day divided into equal doses given every 4–6 hours as needed for cough. Maximum dose 2–6 years: 30 mg/day; 6–12 years: 60 mg/day

Adults: 10–20 mg/dose given every 4–6 hours as needed for cough. Maximum dose 120 mg/day.

Medication Interactions

No major medication interactions have been found with other oral medications.

Adverse Side Effects

Minor: Sedation, drowsiness, dizziness, nausea, constipation, dry mouth, sweating.

Severe: Anxiety, difficulty breathing, awareness of heartbeat, slow heartbeat, rash, sore throat, fever, trembling.

Storage and Administration

The oral medicine should be stored in a cool, dry place away from light. Prolonged exposure to heat, moisture, or light can damage the medicine.

The liquid may be stored at room temperature and does not need to be refrigerated.

If upset stomach occurs, codeine can be given with food or milk.

If the child is unable to swallow the tablet, it can be crushed and mixed with soft food (such as applesauce, pudding, jam, or jelly). This mixture should be swallowed and not chewed. The entire mixture must be swallowed to ensure that the child received the full dose.

Special Instructions

May cause sedation, drowsiness, and dizziness in some people. Until it is known how the child will react to codeine, activities that require mental alertness (such as physical education and playground activity) should be restricted.

May cause dizziness upon standing; therefore, always have the child stand up slowly. If the child becomes dizzy, she should be instructed to sit or lie down immediately.

For older children, dry mouth may be relieved by chewing gum or sucking on hard candy or ice chips. Younger children may need extra liquids.

N o t e s

C romolyn sodium

Gastrocrom
  (capsule)
Intal
  (oral inhaler,
  solution for
  inhalation,
  capsules for
  inhalation)
Nasalcrom
  (nasal spray)
Opticrom
  (eye drops)

Common Uses

Cromolyn sodium is used for a variety of problems. It prevents the release of chemicals in the body that cause allergies and asthma attacks. Cromolyn inhaled into the lungs is used to prevent asthma attacks. Nasal inhalation is used to treat nasal problems due to allergies. Cromolyn eye drops are prescribed to treat and prevent inflammation of the eyelids due to allergies. Oral capsules are used for certain diseases of the intestine and to prevent allergic reactions to food.

Usual Dose

ORAL INHALATION

See the Medication Administration section for instructions on the proper use of an oral inhaler (page 10).

Children older than 5 years and Adults: 2 puffs 4 times a day. For prevention of asthma due to exercise, give 2 puffs just before exercise.

NASAL INHALATION

See the Medication Administration section for instructions on the proper use of a nasal spray (page 15).

Children older than 6 years and Adults: 1 spray into each nostril 3–4 times a day.

SOLUTION FOR INHALATION

See the Medication Administration section for instructions on the proper use of a nebulizer (page 13).

Children older than 2 years and Adults: 20 mg/dose 3–4 times a day.

CAPSULE FOR INHALATION

See the Medication Administration section for instructions on the proper use of a Spinhaler (page 12).

Children older than 5 years and Adults: 1 capsule/dose 4 times a day.

See the Medication Administration section for instructions on the proper technique to instill eye drops (page 8).

Children older than 4 years and Adults: 1–2 drops 4–6 times a day.

ORAL CAPSULES

Children younger than 2 years: 20 mg/kg/day divided into equal doses given 4 times a day. Maximum dose 30 mg/kg/day.

Children 2–12 years: 100 mg/dose given 4 times a day. Maximum dose 40 mg/kg/day.

Children older than 12 years and Adults: 200 mg/dose given 4 times a day. Maximum dose 1600 mg/day.

Medication Interactions

No major medication interactions have been found with other oral medications.

Adverse Side Effects

Minor

ORAL INHALATION AND SOLUTION FOR INHALATION: Cough, wheezing, throat irritation, hoarseness, dizziness, headache, dry mouth, bad taste in the mouth.

CAPSULE FOR INHALATION: Cough, wheezing, throat irritation, hoarseness, dry mouth, bad taste in the mouth.

NASAL INHALATION: Burning of the nasal passages, cough, throat irritation, headache, sneezing, nasal congestion and itching, bad taste in the mouth.

EYE DROPS: Eye stinging, tearing.

ORAL CAPSULES: Dizziness, nausea, vomiting, diarrhea, headache, upset stomach, drowsiness.

Severe: Joint swelling or pain, nosebleeds, nose burning, swelling of face or eyes, rash, swollen glands.

Storage and Administration

The oral medicine should be stored in a cool, dry place away from light. Prolonged exposure to heat, moisture, or light can damage the medicine.

The inhaler should be kept in a cool place. Do not puncture or expose the inhaler to prolonged periods of heat.

The solution and capsules for inhalation should be stored in a cool, dry place away from light. Prolonged exposure to heat, moisture, or light can damage the medicine.

For proper use of the oral medicine, capsules for inhalation, nasal inhaler, nebulizer, or eye drops, read the appropriate medication administration section.

If the child is also taking an orally inhaled bronchodilator (such as albuterol, metaproterenol, or terbutaline), give the entire bronchodilator dose at least 10–15 minutes, or as directed by a physician, before giving cromolyn oral inhalations.

Have the child gargle or rinse his mouth with water to help prevent adverse side effects associated with oral inhalation and solution for inhalation.

Gastrocrom capsules should be mixed with water and taken 30 minutes before a meal. Preparation of the mixture is as follows:

1. Open the capsule(s) and pour into half a glass of hot water. Do not mix with juice, milk, or food.

2. Stir until the solution is clear.

3. Continue stirring and add half a glass of cold water.

4. Have the child drink the entire glass of the mixture.

Special Instructions

Oral inhalations of cromolyn are used to prevent asthma, but they can not treat an asthma attack. When an asthma attack occurs this medicine will not help.

Cyclosporine C

Common Uses

Cyclosporine belongs to the class of medicines called immunosuppressants. Cyclosporine is used to prevent the body from rejecting (not wanting) a new organ, such as a kidney or heart, after transplantation, because it prevents the body's immune system from attacking and destroying the new organ.

Usual Dose

Children and Adults: 3–15 mg/kg/day divided into equal doses given every 12–24 hours.

Medication Interactions

Medications that increase the risk for the development of cyclosporine adverse side effects are:

amiodarone	nicardipine
diltiazem	trimethoprim with sulfamethoxazole
erythromycin	
fluconazole	troleandomycin
ketoconazole	verapamil

Medications that may decrease the effectiveness of cyclosporine are:

phenytoin	sulfamethoxazole
rifabutin	trimethoprim with sulfamethoxazole
rifampin	

Brand Name

Sandimmune (capsule, liquid)

C

Cyclosporine may increase the risk for the development of adverse side effects of:

digoxin

etoposide

A medication that may cause muscle pain, tenderness, or weakness when combined with cyclosporine is:

lovastatin

Adverse Side Effects

Minor: Nausea, vomiting, diarrhea, upset stomach, headache, leg cramps, acne, hair growth.

Severe: Seizures; fever; sore throat; large, painful breasts; tingling of hands or feet; trembling; bleeding; swollen or tender gums; difficult or painful urination; blood in the urine; change in vision; chest pain; irregular heartbeat; unusual bruising or bleeding; yellow skin or eyes; rapid weight gain (3–5 pounds); hearing loss; ringing or buzzing in ear; weakness; difficulty breathing.

Storage and Administration

The oral medicine should be stored in a cool, dry place away from light. Prolonged exposure to heat, moisture, or light can damage the medicine.

The capsule should be swallowed whole with a full glass of water. Do not open it or allow the child to chew it.

The liquid may be stored at room temperature and does not need to be refrigerated.

It is best if cyclosporine is taken on an empty stomach (1 hour before a meal or 2–3 hours after a meal), but if upset stomach occurs it can be given with food or milk.

To improve its taste, mix the cyclosporine liquid in a glass (not plastic) cup with milk, chocolate milk, or orange juice at room temperature. Prepare the mixture just before giving the medicine. Cyclosporine will be damaged if left in the mixture; therefore, do not premix and store. After the child drinks the cyclosporine mixture, refill the glass with the same liquid used (milk, chocolate milk, or orange juice) and have the child drink it.

Special Instructions

If a fever or sore throat occurs notify the child's physician immediately.

It is very important for the child to maintain good dental hygiene. He should visit the dentist regularly.

N o t e s

D esipramine hydrochloride

Brand Names

Norpramin
(tablet)
Pertofrane
(capsule)

Common Uses

Desipramine belongs to the class of medicines called tricyclic antidepressants. Desipramine is used to treat various forms of depression, because it increases the concentration of chemicals in the brain that help counteract the depression.

Usual Dose

Children 6–12 years old: 1–5 mg/kg/day divided into equal doses given more than once a day. Start with the lowest dose and increase according to the physician's directions.

Adolescents: 25–150 mg/day divided into equal doses given as a single or multiple doses. Start with the lowest dose and increase according to the physician's directions.

Adults: 75–300 mg/day divided into equal doses given as a single or multiple doses. Start with the lowest dose and increase according to the physician's directions.

Medication Interactions

Medications that increase the risk for the development of desipramine adverse side effects are:

cimetidine

fluoxetine

Desipramine decreases the effectiveness of:

clonidine

guanethidine

Desipramine increases the risk for the development of bleeding with:

dicumarol

D

Medications that may cause seizures, dangerous increases in body temperature, or death when combined with desipramine are:

isocarboxazid

phenelzine

tranylcypromine

Medications that may increase the risk of sedation, drowsiness, and dizziness when combined with desipramine are:

brompheniramine

chlorpheniramine

diphenhydramine

Adverse Side Effects

Minor: Sedation, drowsiness, dry mouth, constipation, fatigue, bad taste in the mouth, insomnia, dizziness, increased sensitivity to sunlight, nervousness, anxiety, sweating, nausea, vomiting.

Severe: Blurred vision; confusion; seizures; chest pain; fever; sore throat; hallucinations; irregular heartbeat; stomach pain; loss of balance; unusual bruising or bleeding; yellow skin or eyes; joint pain; swollen breasts; trembling; unintentional movements of the face, mouth, and tongue.

Storage and Administration

The oral medicine should be stored in a cool, dry place away from light. Prolonged exposure to heat, moisture, or light can damage the medicine.

If upset stomach occurs, desipramine can be given with food or milk.

If the child is unable to swallow pills, the tablets can be crushed or the capsule opened and mixed with a small amount of water or soft food (such as applesauce, pudding, jam, or jelly). This mixture should be swallowed and not chewed. The entire mixture must be swallowed to ensure that the child received the full dose.

Special Instructions

May cause sedation, drowsiness, and dizziness in some people. Until it is known how the child will react to the medicine, activities that require mental alertness (such as physical education and playground activity) should be restricted.

D

May cause dizziness upon standing; therefore, always have the child stand up slowly. If the child becomes dizzy, he should be instructed to sit or lie down immediately.

In children with a seizure disorder, this medicine may cause seizures even if the child's condition is currently controlled.

For older children, dry mouth may be relieved by chewing gum or sucking on hard candy or ice chips. Younger children may need extra liquids.

Avoid prolonged exposure to sunlight because this medication may cause the child to be more sensitive to it.

Desipramine increases the chance of heat stroke because it decreases the child's ability to sweat; therefore, physical education and playground activity should be restricted, especially on hot days.

Do not allow the child to abruptly stop taking this medicine. Suddenly stopping the medicine can cause nausea, headache, upset stomach, fatigue, or depression.

N o t e s

Dexamethasone

Common Uses

Dexamethasone belongs to the class of medicines called corticosteroids. Oral inhalation of the medicine is used to treat asthma. Nasal inhalation is used to provide relief of stuffy nose, nasal irritation, and discomfort due to hay fever and allergies. Oral tablets, liquids, and concentrates are used to treat asthma, allergies, inflammatory diseases, and various other problems. Skin creams and aerosols are used to relieve the itching, redness, and discomfort of various skin diseases and rashes caused by poison oak and poison ivy. Eye drops and ointment are used to treat inflammation of the eye caused by allergies or various other problems. Dexamethasone is effective because it affects many different substances in the body that may cause or worsen these conditions.

Usual Dose

EYE DROPS AND OINTMENT

See the Medication Administration section for instructions on the proper use of ophthalmic medications (page 8).

Children and Adults

DROPS: Start with 1–2 drops every 1 hour during the day and every 2 hours during the night, then adjust the dose as instructed by the physician to a final dosing frequency of 3 times a day.

OINTMENT: Apply as directed to the lower eyelid 3–4 times a day.

ORAL INHALATION

See the Medication Administration section for instructions on the proper use of an oral inhaler (page 10).

Children: 2 inhalations 3–4 times a day. Maximum dose 8 inhalations/day.

Adults: 3 inhalations 3–4 times a day. Maximum dose 12 inhalations/day.

Brand Names

Aeroseb–Dex
(skin aerosol)

AK–Dex
(eye drops,
eye ointment)

Decadron
(eye drops,
eye ointment,
tablet, liquid,
skin cream)

Decadron
Respihaler
(oral inhaler)

Decadron
Turbinaire
(nasal inhaler)

Decaspray
(skin aerosol)

Dexameth
(tablet)

Dexamethasone
Intensol
(concentrate)

Dexone
(tablet)

Hexadrol
(tablet, liquid)

Maxidex
(eye drops,
eye ointment)

D

See the Medication Administration section for instructions on the proper use of a nasal inhaler (page 16).

Children 6–12 years old: 1–2 sprays in each nostril twice a day. Maximum dose 8 sprays in each nostril/day.

Children older than 12 years and Adults: 2 sprays in each nostril 2–3 times a day. Maximum dose 12 sprays in each nostril/day.

TABLET, LIQUID, AND CONCENTRATE

Children: 0.08–0.3 mg/kg/day divided into equal doses given every 6–12 hours.

Adults: 0.75–9 mg/day divided into equal doses given every 6–12 hours.

SKIN CREAM AND AEROSOL

Children and Adults: Apply as directed by the physician to the infected area 2–4 times a day.

Medication Interactions

A medication that may increase the risk for the development of dexamethasone adverse side effects is:

troleandomycin

Medications that may decrease the effectiveness of dexamethasone are:

phenobarbital   primidone

phenytoin   rifampin

Dexamethasone decreases the effectiveness of:

aspirin   phenytoin

bismuth subsalicylate   salsalate

choline salicylate   sodium salicylate

magnesium salicylate

Adverse Side Effects

Minor

EYE DROPS AND OINTMENT: Temporary burning or stinging; temporary blurred vision.

ORAL INHALATION: Fungal growth in the mouth, hoarseness, dry mouth, bad taste in the mouth, cough, headache, dizziness.

NASAL INHALATION: Irritation and burning of the nose, sneezing, fungal growth in nose, stuffy or runny nose, bad taste in the mouth, headache, dizziness.

TABLET AND LIQUID: Round face, weight gain, acne, upset stomach, nausea, vomiting, increased appetite, dizziness.

SKIN MEDICINE: Acne, dry skin, mild burning or stinging sensation, itching, minor rash.

Severe: Rash; hives; skin blistering; loss of skin color; skin infection at the site where the medicine is used; difficulty swallowing; increased thirst; headache; seizures; insomnia; fatigue; abnormal hair growth; black, tarry stools; sore throat; fever; hallucinations; irregular heartbeat; persistent burning or stinging of the eye; blurred vision or halos around light; stomach pain; nightmares; difficulty breathing; unusual weakness; leg cramping.

Storage and Administration

The oral medicine should be stored in a cool, dry place away from light. Prolonged exposure to heat, moisture, or light can damage the medicine.

The inhaler should be kept in a cool place. Do not puncture or expose the inhaler to prolonged periods of heat.

The liquid and concentrate may be stored at room temperature and do not need to be refrigerated.

The skin cream and aerosol may be stored at room temperature.

The concentrate should be mixed with half a cup or more of fruit juice, milk, water, carbonated beverage, or a small amount of soft food (such as applesauce, pudding, jam, or jelly). Prepare the mixture just before giving the dose. Dexamethasone will be damaged if left in the mixture; therefore, do not premix and store.

D

For proper use of the eye medication or the oral or nasal inhaler read the appropriate medication administration section.

If the child is also taking an orally inhaled bronchodilator (such as albuterol, metaproterenol, or terbutaline) give the entire broncho-dilator dose at least 10–15 minutes, or as directed by a physician, before giving dexamethasone oral inhalations.

After oral inhalation, have the child rinse his mouth with water. This helps prevent some of the side effects associated with oral inhalation.

It is best to have the child take this medicine with food or milk to decrease or prevent stomach upset.

If the child is unable to swallow the tablet, it can be crushed and mixed with soft food (such as applesauce, pudding, jam, or jelly). This mixture should be swallowed and not chewed. The entire mixture must be swallowed to ensure that the child received the full dose.

Special Instructions

May cause dizziness in some people. Until it is known how the child will react to the medicine, activities that require mental alertness (such as physical education and playground activity) should be restricted.

For older children, dry mouth may be relieved by chewing gum or sucking on hard candy or ice chips. Younger children may need extra liquids.

Oral inhalations of dexamethasone are used to prevent asthma, but it can not treat an asthma attack. When an asthma attack occurs this medicine will not help.

If the child has been taking dexamethasone for more than 1 week, do not abruptly stop it. Suddenly stopping the oral medicine (tablet, liquid, or concentrate) can cause nausea, vomiting, weakness, fever, shortness of breath, stomach or back pain, or dizziness.

If the child has been taking this medicine for more than 1 week, notify the physician who prescribed the dexamethasone if a serious injury or illness occurs.

Skin cream and skin aerosol are to be used only on the skin. Be careful not to get them into the child's eyes.

D

Tight-fitting diapers should not be used when the skin medicine is being applied to the diaper area.

The child's physician should be notified if black, tarry stools occur.

N o t e s

D extroamphetamine

Brand Names

Dexedrine
(tablet, liquid)
Dexedrine
Spansules
(long-acting
capsule)
Ferndex
(tablet)
Spancap No. 1
(long-acting
capsule)

Common Uses

Dextroamphetamine belongs to the class of medicines called stimulants, which are used to treat narcolepsy and attention deficit disorder with hyperactivity (ADDH). Dextroamphetamine is able to treat these conditions because it causes chemicals to be released into the brain, which allows more focused attention.

Usual Dose

NARCOLEPSY

Children 6–12 years old: Start with 5 mg/day; increase the dose according to the physician's directions until the desired effect is obtained. Maximum dose 60 mg/day.

Children older than 12 years and Adults: Start with 10 mg/day; increase the dose according to the physician's directions until the desired effect is obtained. Maximum dose 60 mg/day.

ATTENTION DEFICIT DISORDER WITH HYPERACTIVITY

Children 3–5 years old: 2.5–40 mg/day divided into equal doses given 1–2 times a day.

Children older than 5 years: 5–40 mg/day divided into equal doses given 1–2 times a day.

Medication Interactions

Medications that increase the risk for the development of dextroamphetamine adverse side effects are:

furazolidone   sodium bicarbonate

potassium citrate   sodium citrate

sodium acetate   sodium lactate

Medications that may cause dangerous increases in body temperature, brain hemorrhage, seizures, or death when combined with dextroamphetamine are:

isocarboxazid   phenelzine

pargyline   tranylcypromine

Adverse Side Effects

Minor: Constipation, upset stomach, nausea, diarrhea, dizziness, dry mouth, insomnia, irritability, loss of appetite, hyperactivity, bad taste in the mouth, nervousness.

Severe: Blurred vision; confusion; fatigue; headache; awareness of heartbeat; rapid heartbeat; rash; hives, sweating; chest pain; trembling; uncontrolled movements of head, arms, or legs.

Storage and Administration

The oral medicine should be stored in a cool, dry place away from light. Prolonged exposure to heat, moisture, or light can damage the medicine.

The liquid may be stored at room temperature and does not need to be refrigerated.

It is best to give dextroamphetamine with food or milk to decrease or prevent stomach upset.

Dextroamphetamine tablets usually are given 2–3 times a day; the long-acting capsule usually can be given once a day.

The long-acting capsule should be swallowed whole with a full glass of water. Do not crush or allow the child to chew it.

Special Instructions

May cause dizziness in some people. Until it is known how the child will react to the medicine, activities that require mental alertness (such as physical education and playground activity) should be restricted.

For older children, dry mouth may be relieved by chewing gum or sucking on hard candy or ice chips. Younger children may need extra liquids.

Have the child avoid drinking beverages containing caffeine and eating excessive amounts of chocolate because this may make her susceptible to insomnia, irritability, and hyperactivity.

D extromethorphan

Brand Names

Benylin DM
(liquid)

Children's Hold
(lozenge)

Delsym (long-
acting liquid)

Hold DM
(lozenge)

Pertussin CS
(liquid)

Pertussin ES
(liquid)

Robitussin
Cough
Calmers
(lozenge)

Robitussin
Pediatric
(liquid)

Scot-Tussin DM
(lozenge)

St. Joseph
Cough
Suppressant
(liquid)

Sucrets Cough
Control
(lozenge)

Vicks Formula
44
(liquid)

Vicks Formula
44 Pediatric
Formula
(liquid)

Common Uses

Dextromethorphan belongs to the class of medicines called antitussives. Dextromethorphan is used to relieve coughs caused by common colds and other respiratory infections, because it suppresses the urge to cough.

Usual Dose

LIQUID AND LOZENGE*

Children 2–5 years old: 2.5–7.5 mg/dose given every 4–8 hours. Maximum dose 30 mg/day.

Children 6–12 years old: 5–10 mg/dose given every 4 hours or 15 mg/dose every 6–8 hours. Maximum dose 60 mg/day.

Children older than 12 years and Adults: 10–30 mg/dose given every 4–8 hours. Maximum dose 120 mg/day.

*The use of lozenges in young children is not recommended because of the possibility of choking.

LONG-ACTING LIQUID

Children 2–5 years old: 15 mg/dose given every 12 hours.

Children 6–12 years old: 30 mg/dose given every 12 hours.

Children older than 12 years and Adults: 60 mg/dose given every 12 hours.

Medication Interactions

No major medication interactions have been found with other oral medications.

Adverse Side Effects

Minor: Drowsiness, upset stomach.

Severe: Confusion, nervousness, rash, stomach pain, diarrhea, weakness.

Storage and Administration

The oral medicine should be stored in a cool, dry place away from light. Prolonged exposure to heat, moisture, or light can damage the medicine.

The liquid may be stored at room temperature and does not need to be refrigerated.

If upset stomach occurs, dextromethorphan can be given with food.

Special Instructions

May cause drowsiness in some people. Until it is known how the child will react to the medicine, activities that require mental alertness (such as physical education and playground activity) should be restricted.

N o t e s

D icloxacillin sodium

Brand Names

Dycill
(capsule)
Dynapen
(capsule,
liquid)
Pathocil
(capsule,
liquid)

Common Uses

Dicloxacillin belongs to the class of medicines called antibiotics, which are used to treat a variety of bacterial infections. Dicloxacillin is prescribed for infections of the respiratory tract, skin, soft tissue, and bones, because it prevents the bacteria from growing.

Dicloxacillin is effective only against bacterial infections, not those caused by viruses, parasites, or yeast.

Usual Dose

Children who weigh less than 40 kg (88 lb): 12.5–100 mg/kg/day divided into equal doses given every 6 hours.

Children who weigh more than 40 kg and Adults: 125–500 mg/dose given every 6 hours.

Medication Interactions

Medications that decrease the effectiveness of dicloxacillin are:

demeclocycline	minocycline
doxycycline	oxytetracycline
methacycline	tetracycline

Adverse Side Effects

Minor: Diarrhea, nausea, vomiting, heartburn, upset stomach, darkened tongue.

Severe: Rash, hives, difficulty breathing, blood in the urine, sore throat, fever, stomach cramps, seizures, unexplained bleeding or bruising, severe diarrhea.

Storage and Administration

The oral medicine should be stored in a cool, dry place away from light. Prolonged exposure to heat, moisture, or light can damage the medicine.

Before measuring the dose, the liquid form of dicloxacillin should be shaken well. Refrigeration of the liquid is recommended. After receiving the liquid medicine from the pharmacy, it is good only for 14 days; therefore, always check the expiration date on the prescription label before using.

Dicloxacillin works best when taken on an empty stomach (1 hour before a meal or 2–3 hours after a meal).

If the child is unable to swallow the capsule, it can be opened and mixed with a small amount of water. The entire mixture must be swallowed to ensure that the child received the full dose.

Special Instructions

The child's physician should be notified if the infection worsens or does not improve within 3–5 days.

N o t e s

D idanosine

Brand Name

Videx
(chewable
tablet,
powder,
liquid)

Common Uses

Didanosine belongs to the class of medicines called antivirals. Different antivirals are prescribed to treat different viral infections. Didanosine is used to treat children infected with HIV, the virus that causes AIDS, because it prevents the virus from growing.

Didanosine is effective only against the HIV virus, not other viruses, bacteria, parasites, or yeast.

Usual Dose

TABLET*

Children who weigh less than 35 kg (77 lb): 100–300 mg/m²/day divided into equal doses given every 12 hours.

Children who weigh more than 35 kg and Adults:

35–49 kg (77–108 lb): 125 mg/dose given every 12 hours.

50–74 kg (110–163 lb): 200 mg/dose given every 12 hours.

75 kg (165 lb) or more: 300 mg/dose given every 12 hours.

*Children younger than 1 year should be given the dose in 1 tablet. Children older than 1 year should be given the dose in 2 tablets.

LIQUID

Children who weigh less than 35 kg: 100–300 mg/m²/day divided into equal doses given every 12 hours.

POWDER

Children who weigh more than 35 kg and Adults:

35–49 kg: 167 mg/dose every 12 hours.

50–74 kg: 250 mg/dose every 12 hours.

75 kg or more: 375 mg/dose every 12 hours.

Medication Interactions

A medication that may decrease the effectiveness of didanosine is:

dapsone

Didanosine may decrease the effectiveness of:

ciprofloxacin   norfloxacin

enoxacin   ofloxacin

lomefloxacin

Adverse Side Effects

Minor: Headache, dizziness, insomnia, nervousness, diarrhea, upset stomach, dry mouth, bad taste in the mouth.

Severe: Nausea, vomiting, stomach pain, numbness, tingling or pain in the hands or feet, seizures, yellow skin or eyes, muscle or joint pain.

Storage and Administration

The oral medicine should be stored in a cool, dry place away from light. Prolonged exposure to heat, moisture, or light can damage the medicine.

Before measuring the dose, the liquid form of didanosine should be shaken well. Refrigeration of the liquid is recommended. After receiving the liquid medicine from the pharmacy, it is good only for 30 days; therefore, always check the expiration date on the prescription label before using.

Should be taken on an empty stomach (1 hour before a meal or 2–3 hours after a meal).

The chewable tablet should be chewed thoroughly before swallowing. If the child cannot, or will not chew the tablet, it can be crushed and placed in water. Two tablets can be placed in 1 ounce of water. Stir until the tablets are well dispersed (they will not completely dissolve), then have the child drink it immediately. The mixture is stable only for 1 hour at room temperature; therefore, do not save it. Do not substitute acid-containing beverages (such as fruit juice) for water. Acid-containing beverages can damage the medicine.

The didanosine powder should be mixed with 4 ounces of water before being swallowed. Stir until the powder is dissolved and then

D

have the child drink it immediately. The mixture is stable only for 4 hours at room temperature; therefore, do not save it. Do not substitute acid-containing beverages (such as fruit juice) for water. Acid-containing beverages can damage the medicine.

The child should not drink acid-containing beverages from 1 hour before to 2–3 hours after taking didanosine.

Special Instructions

May cause dizziness in some people. Until it is known how the child will react to didanosine, activities that require mental alertness (such as physical education and playground activity) should be restricted.

Report any vomiting, stomach pain, numbness, tingling, or pain in the hands or feet to the child's physician immediately.

N o t e s

Digoxin D

Common Uses

Digoxin belongs to the class of medicines called antiarrhythmics. Digoxin is used to strengthen the heartbeat and make it beat in a regular rate and rhythm, because it changes the amount of sodium, potassium, and calcium in the heart.

Usual Dose

Children 1–24 months old: 10–15 mcg/kg/day divided into equal doses given every 12 hours.

Children 2–5 years: 7.5–10 mcg/kg/day divided into equal doses given every 12 hours.

Children 5–10 years: 5–10 mcg/kg/day divided into equal doses given every 12 hours.

Children older than 10 years: 2.5–5 mcg/kg/dose given once a day.

Adults: 125–500 mcg/dose given once a day.

Medication Interactions

Medications that may increase the risk for the development of digoxin adverse side effects are:

amiodarone	indomethacin
bepridil	methacycline
bumetanide	methimazole*
chlorothiazide	minocycline
cyclosporine	oxytetracycline
demeclocycline	propylthiouracil*
doxycycline	quinidine
erythromycin	quinine
ethacrynic acid	tetracycline
furosemide	verapamil
hydrochlorothiazide	

Brand Names

Lanoxicaps
(capsule)

Lanoxin
(tablet, liquid)

D

Medications that may decrease the effectiveness of digoxin are:

antacids	liothyronine*
cholestyramine	liotrix*
colestipol	metoclopramide
dextrothyroxine*	thyroglobulin*
levothyroxine*	thyroid*

*These interactions depend on how well the thyroid disease is controlled and if these medications were started before or after digoxin.

Adverse Side Effects

Minor: Nausea, diarrhea, headache, temporary drowsiness or fatigue, weakness.

Severe: Disorientation, hallucinations, loss of appetite, vomiting, severe abdominal pain, awareness of heartbeat, slow heartbeat, unusual or irregular heartbeat, blurred vision, yellow or green vision, vision with halos around objects, persistent headache, persistent drowsiness or fatigue, skin rash, muscle weakness, depression.

Storage and Administration

The oral medicine should be stored in a cool, dry place away from light. Prolonged exposure to heat, moisture, or light can damage the medicine.

The liquid may be stored at room temperature and does not need to be refrigerated.

If upset stomach occurs, digoxin can be given with food.

Do not allow the child to take antacids within 1 hour before or 2 hours after taking digoxin.

If the child is unable to swallow the pills, the tablet can be crushed and the capsule can be opened and mixed with water or soft food (such as applesauce, pudding, jam, or jelly). This mixture should be swallowed and not chewed. The entire mixture must be swallowed to ensure that the child received the full dose.

Special Instructions

Digoxin may cause drowsiness in some people. Until it is known how the child will react to the medicine, activities that require mental alertness (such as physical education and playground activity) should be restricted.

Have the child avoid drinking beverages containing caffeine or eating excessive amounts of chocolate, because these may cause irregular heartbeats to occur.

N o t e s

D iphenhydramine hydrochloride

Brand Names

AllerMax
  Caplets
  (tablet)
Banophen
  (capsule)
Banophen
  Caplets
  (tablet)
Belix
  (liquid)
Benadryl
  (capsule,
  liquid)
Benadryl 25
  (capsule,
  tablet)
Benylin Cough
  (liquid)
Dormarex 2
  (tablet)
Genahist
  (tablet, liquid)
Hydramine
  (liquid)
Phendry
  (liquid)
Tusstat
  (liquid)

Common Uses

Diphenhydramine belongs to the class of medicines called antihistamines. Diphenhydramine is used to treat children with seasonal and constant runny nose and sneezing caused by allergies and colds, because it blocks the chemical histamine, which causes these problems. Diphenhydramine also is used to prevent motion sickness, and to make children and adults sleepy.

Usual Dose

Children who weigh more than 10 kg (22 lb): 5 mg/kg/day divided into equal doses given every 6–8 hours or 12.5–25 mg/dose every 6–8 hours. Maximum dose 300 mg/day.

Adults: 25–50 mg/dose every 6–8 hours.

Medication Interactions

Medications that may increase the risk of sedation, drowsiness, and dizziness when combined with diphenhydramine are:

alcohol	fluphenazine
amitriptyline	nortriptyline
amoxapine	perphenazine
clomipramine	prochlorperazine
desipramine	thioridazine
doxepin	trifluoperazine

Adverse Side Effects

Minor: Drowsiness; dizziness; sedation; dry mouth, nose and throat; nausea; headache; upset stomach; sweating; constipation; increased sensitivity to sunlight.

Severe: Sore throat, fever, unusual bruising or bleeding, rash, clumsiness, hallucinations, fast heartbeat, awareness of heartbeat, seizures, difficulty breathing, chest tightness, weakness, fatigue, blurred vision.

Storage and Administration

The oral medicine should be stored in a cool, dry place away from light. Prolonged exposure to heat, moisture, or light can damage the medicine.

The liquid may be stored at room temperature and does not need to be refrigerated.

If upset stomach occurs, diphenhydramine can be given with food or milk.

If the child is unable to swallow pills, the tablet can be crushed or the capsules opened and mixed with a small amount of water or soft food (such as applesauce, pudding, jam, or jelly). This mixture should be swallowed and not chewed. The entire mixture must be swallowed to ensure that the child received the full dose.

Special Instructions

May cause sedation, drowsiness, and dizziness in some people. Until it is known how the child will react to the medicine, activities that require mental alertness (such as physical education and playground activity) should be restricted.

May cause dizziness upon standing; therefore, always have the child stand up slowly. If the child becomes dizzy, she should be instructed to sit or lie down immediately.

In children with a seizure disorder, this medication may cause seizures even if the seizures are currently controlled.

For older children, dry mouth may be relieved by chewing gum or sucking on hard candy or ice chips. Younger children may need extra liquids

Avoid prolonged exposure to sunlight because this medication may cause the child to be more sensitive to it.

D ivalproex sodium

Brand Name

Depakote
(enteric-
coated tablet,
sprinkle
capsule)

Common Uses

Divalproex sodium belongs to the class of medicines called anticonvulsants. Divalproex sodium is used to treat and control seizures, because it helps prevent the spread of the seizure throughout the brain.

Usual Dose

Children and Adults: 10–60 mg/kg/day divided into equal doses given 1–3 times a day.

Medication Interactions

A medication that may decrease the effectiveness of divalproex sodium is:

carbamazepine

Divalproex sodium may increase the risk for the development of adverse side effects of:

carbamazepine

Adverse Side Effects

Minor: Nausea, vomiting, diarrhea, upset stomach, drowsiness, trembling, headache, constipation, weakness.

Severe: Unusual bruising or bleeding, rash, yellow skin or eyes, double vision, unusual eye movements, swelling of the feet and legs.

Storage and Administration

The oral medicine should be stored in a cool, dry place away from light. Prolonged exposure to heat, moisture, or light can damage the medicine.

If upset stomach occurs, divalproex sodium can be given with food.

The enteric-coated tablet should be swallowed whole with a full glass of water. Do not crush or allow the child to chew it.

Sprinkle capsules can be swallowed whole or opened and sprinkled over soft food (such as applesauce, pudding, jam, or jelly). This mixture should be swallowed and not chewed. The entire mixture must be swallowed to ensure that the child received the full dose. The medicine will be damaged if left in the mixture; therefore, do not premix and store.

Special Instructions

May cause sedation, drowsiness, and dizziness in some people. Until it is known how the child will react to the medicine, activities that require mental alertness (such as physical education and playground activity) should be restricted.

Do not suddenly stop giving divalproex sodium to the child unless instructed to do so by a physician. Suddenly stopping this medication may cause severe seizures to occur.

N o t e s

D oxycycline

Brand Names

Doryx
(capsule)

Doxy Caps
(capsule)

Doxychel
Hyclate
(capsule,
tablet)

Vibramycin
(capsule,
liquid)

Vibra-Tabs
(tablet)

Common Uses

Doxycycline belongs to the class of medicines called antibiotics, which are used to treat a variety of bacterial infections. Doxycycline is prescribed for infections of the urinary and respiratory tract, because it prevents the bacteria from growing.

Doxycycline is effective only against bacterial infections, not those caused by viruses, parasites, or yeast.

Usual Dose

Children 8 years old and older: 2–5 mg/kg/day divided into equal doses given every 12–24 hours. Maximum dose 200 mg/day.

Children more than 45 kg (100 lb) and Adults: 100–200 mg/day divided into equal doses given every 12–24 hours.

Medication Interactions

Medications that may decrease the effectiveness of doxycycline are:

antacids	penicillin G
amoxicillin	penicillin V
ampicillin	phenobarbital
bismuth salts	phenytoin
carbamazepine	potassium citrate
cloxacillin	primidone
dicloxacillin	sodium acetate
iron salts	sodium bicarbonate
nafcillin	sodium citrate
oxacillin	sodium lactate

Doxycycline increases the risk for the development of adverse side effects of:

digoxin

methoxyflurane

Adverse Side Effects

Minor: Nausea, diarrhea, dizziness, upset stomach, vomiting, increased sensitivity to sunlight, tooth discoloration in children who do not yet have their permanent teeth.

Severe: Difficulty breathing, joint pain, rash, sore throat, fever, yellow skin or eyes, blurred vision.

Storage and Administration

The oral medicine should be stored in a cool, dry place away from light. Prolonged exposure to heat, moisture, or light can damage the medicine.

Before the dose is measured, the liquid form of doxycycline should be shaken well. The liquid may be stored at room temperature and does not need to be refrigerated. After receiving the liquid medicine from the pharmacy, it is good only for 14 days; therefore, always check the expiration date on the prescription label before using.

Doxycycline works best when taken on an empty stomach (1 hour before a meal or 2–3 hours after a meal), but if upset stomach occurs it can be given with food or milk.

The tablets and capsules should be given with a full glass of water.

If the child is unable to swallow pills, the tablets can be crushed or the capsules opened and mixed with a small amount of water, carbonated beverage, or soft food (such as applesauce, pudding, jam, or jelly). This mixture should be swallowed and not chewed. The entire mixture must be swallowed to ensure that the child received the full dose.

Do not allow the child to take antacids within 2 hours before or 2 hours after taking doxycycline.

D

Special Instructions

The child's physician should be notified if the infection worsens or does not improve within 3–5 days.

Have the child avoid prolonged exposure to sunlight because this medication causes her to be more sensitive to it.

Irreversible tooth discoloration may occur in the unerupted permanent teeth of children who do not have all their permanent teeth.

N o t e s

Enalapril maleate E

Common Uses

Enalapril belongs to the class of medicines called angiotensin-converting enzyme inhibitors (ACE inhibitors). Enalapril is used to treat and control high blood pressure and weak hearts, because it blocks angiotensin-converting enzyme from producing angiotensin II, a chemical that causes blood vessels to narrow.

Usual Doses

Infants and Children: 0.1–0.43 mg/kg/day given 1–2 times a day.

Adults: 2.5–40 mg/day divided into equal doses given 1–2 times a day.

Medication Interactions

A medication that may decrease the effectiveness of enalapril is:

indomethacin

Adverse Side Effects

Minor: Nausea, vomiting, diarrhea, upset stomach, dizziness, drowsiness, fatigue, insomnia, nervousness, cough, sweating, loss of taste.

Severe: Chest pain; difficulty swallowing or breathing; fainting; fever; sore throat or mouth; hoarseness; rash; muscle weakness or cramps; swelling of the hands, feet, face, tongue, lips, or eyes; awareness of heartbeat; irregular heartbeat; numbness or tingling in fingers or toes; yellow skin or eyes.

Storage and Administration

The oral medicine should be stored in a cool, dry place away from light. Prolonged exposure to heat, moisture, or light can damage the medicine.

If upset stomach occurs, the medicine can be given with food, water, milk, or juice.

Brand Name

Vasotec
(tablet)

E

If the child is unable to swallow the enalapril tablet, it can be crushed and mixed with a small amount of water, juice, or soft food (such as applesauce, pudding, jam, or jelly). This mixture should be swallowed and not chewed. The entire mixture must be swallowed to ensure that the child received the full dose.

Special Instructions

May cause drowsiness or dizziness in some people. Until it is known how the child will react to the medicine, activities that require mental alertness (such as physical education and playground activity) should be restricted.

May cause dizziness upon standing; therefore, always have the child stand up slowly. If the child becomes dizzy, she should be instructed to sit or lie down immediately.

N o t e s

Epinephrine

Common Uses

Epinephrine belongs to the class of medicines called bronchodilators. Inhaled epinephrine is used to treat and prevent asthma attacks and improve breathing difficulties caused by various other non–infection-related respiratory problems. Epinephrine is effective in these conditions because it opens the airways and prevents them from closing again. Injected epineph-rine is used to prevent and treat problems associated with a severe allergic reaction, because it blocks the chemical histamine, which causes these reactions.

Usual Dose

ORAL INHALATION

See the Medication Administration section for instructions on the proper use of an oral inhaler (page 10).

Children older than 4 years and Adults: 1–2 inhalations every 3 hours as needed for wheezing and shortness of breath.

SOLUTION FOR INHALATION

See the Medication Administration section for instructions on the proper use of a nebulizer (page 13).

Infants and Children: 0.25–0.5 mL of racemic epi-nephrine (AsthmaNefrin and Vaponefrin) diluted with 3 mL of normal saline and given every 1–4 hours.

AUTO-INJECTOR

Children: 0.15–0.3 mg injected once as instructed by a physician, nurse, or pharmacist.

Adults: 0.3 mg injected once as instructed by a physician, nurse, or pharmacist.

Medication Interactions

No major medication interactions have been found with other oral medications.

Brand Names

AsthmaHaler Mist
(oral inhaler)

AsthmaNefrin
(solution for inhalation)

Bronitin Mist
(oral inhaler)

Bronkaid Mist
(oral inhaler)

Epipen
(prefilled auto-injector)

Epipen Jr.
(prefilled auto-injector)

Medihaler-Epi
(oral inhaler)

Primatene Mist
(oral inhaler)

Vaponefrin
(solution for inhalation)

E

Adverse Side Effects

Minor

ORAL INHALATION: Dry throat and mouth. The following side effects mainly occur when too many inhalations are given or when the medicine is given too often: nervousness, headache, fast heartbeat, trembling, insomnia, increased blood pressure, dizziness, nausea, vomiting, hyperactivity, flushing, upset stomach.

SOLUTION FOR INHALATION: Nervousness, hyperactivity, headache, fast heartbeat, trembling, insomnia, increased blood pressure, dizziness, upset stomach, nausea, vomiting, flushing.

INJECTED: Nausea, vomiting, fast heartbeat, sweating, dizziness, headache, nervousness, trembling, increased blood pressure. If these continue for an extended period of time, contact the child's physician.

Severe: Chest pain, hallucinations, difficult or painful urination, rash, irregular heartbeat, difficulty breathing, weakness.

Storage and Administration

The inhaler should be kept in a cool place. Do not puncture the inhaler or expose it to prolonged periods of heat.

The solution for inhalation and auto-injector should be stored in a cool, dry place away from light. Prolonged exposure to heat, moisture, or light can damage the medicine.

For proper use of the inhaler or nebulizer, read the appropriate medication administration section.

To prevent dry throat and mouth, have the child rinse his mouth with water after each inhalation.

If the child is receiving more than 1 puff of epinephrine, give the second puff at least 1 minute after the first one.

If the child is receiving another inhaled medicine for asthma, the entire epinephrine dose should be given at least 10–15 minutes before the other inhaled medicine is given, or as directed by a physician.

Special Instructions

Consult the child's physician about giving extra inhalations, because increasing the number of inhalations may be dangerous.

After using the prefilled auto-injector contact the child's physician for further instructions.

Erythromycin base

Common Uses

Erythromycin base belongs to the class of medicines called antibiotics, which are used to treat a variety of bacterial infections. Erythromycin base is prescribed for infections of the middle ear and respiratory tract, because it prevents the bacteria from growing.

Erythromycin base is effective only against bacterial infections, not those caused by viruses, parasites, or yeast.

Usual Dose

Infants and Children: 30–50 mg/kg/day divided into equal doses given every 6–8 hours. Maximum dose 2 g/day.

Adults: 250–500 mg/dose given every 6–12 hours.

Medication Interactions

Erythromycin base may increase the risk for the development of adverse side effects of:

astemizole	methylprednisolone
carbamazepine	terfenadine
digoxin	theophylline
loratadine	warfarin

Adverse Side Effects

Minor: Nausea, vomiting, diarrhea, upset stomach, sore mouth, fatigue, darkened tongue.

Severe: Rash, fever, hives, stomach pain or cramps, hearing loss, yellow skin or eyes.

Storage and Administration

The oral medicine should be stored in a cool, dry place away from light. Prolonged exposure to heat, moisture, or light can damage the medicine.

Brand Names

E-Mycin
  (enteric-
  coated tablet)
Eryc
  (long-acting
  capsule,
  enteric-
  coated
  capsule)
Ery-Tab
  (enteric-
  coated tablet)
PCE Dispertab
  (tablet)
Robimycin
  (enteric-
  coated tablet)

E

Erythromycin base works best when taken on an empty stomach (1 hour before a meal or 2–3 hours after a meal). Certain brands of erythromycin base may be taken with food. Check with the child's physician or a pharmacist to see if this prescription may be taken with food.

The long-acting capsule, enteric-coated tablet, and enteric-coated capsule should be swallowed whole with a full glass of water. Do not crush or allow the child to chew it.

If the child is unable to swallow the nonchewable tablet, it can be crushed and mixed with water or soft food (such as applesauce, pudding, jam, or jelly). This mixture should be swallowed and not chewed. The entire mixture must be swallowed to ensure that the child received the entire dose.

Do not allow the child to drink fruit juice for 1 hour before or 1 hour after taking this medicine.

Special Instructions

The child's physician should be notified if the infection worsens or does not improve within 3–5 days.

N o t e s

Erythromycin estolate

Common Uses

Erythromycin estolate belongs to the class of medicines called antibiotics, which are used to treat a variety of bacterial infections. Erythromycin estolate is prescribed for infections of the middle ear and respiratory tract, because it prevents the bacteria from growing.

Erythromycin estolate is effective only against bacterial infections, not those caused by viruses, parasites, or yeast.

Usual Dose

Infants and Children: 30–50 mg/kg/day divided into equal doses and given every 8–12 hours. Maximum dose 2 g/day.

Adults: 250–500 mg/dose given every 6–12 hours.

Medication Interactions

Erythromycin estolate may increase the risk for the development of adverse side effects of:

astemizole	methylprednisolone
bromocriptine	terfenadine
carbamazepine	theophylline
digoxin	warfarin
loratadine	

Adverse Side Effects

Minor: Nausea, vomiting, diarrhea, upset stomach, sore mouth, fatigue, darkened tongue.

Severe: Rash, fever, hives, stomach pain or cramps, hearing loss, yellow skin or eyes.

Brand Name

Ilosone
(tablet,
capsule,
liquid)

E

Storage and Administration

The oral medicine should be stored in a cool, dry place away from light. Prolonged exposure to heat, moisture, or light can damage the medicine.

Before the dose is measured, the liquid form of erythromycin estolate should be shaken well. Refrigeration of the liquid is recommended to preserve its taste. After receiving the liquid medicine from the pharmacy, it is good only for 14 days; therefore, always check the expiration date on the prescription label before using.

If the liquid comes in a dropper bottle, double check the instructions on the label. Some oral solutions come in dropper bottles, and may cause harm if applied to the eye or ear.

The tablet and capsule should be taken with a full glass of water.

If the child is unable to swallow the pills, the tablets can be crushed or the capsules opened and mixed with water, fruit juice, carbonated beverage, or soft food (such as applesauce, pudding, jam, or jelly). This mixture should be swallowed and not chewed. The entire mixture must be swallowed to ensure that the child received the entire dose.

If upset stomach occurs, the medicine can be given with food or milk.

Special Instructions

The child's physician should be notified if the infection worsens or does not improve within 3–5 days.

N o t e s

Erythromycin ethylsuccinate

Common Uses

Erythromycin ethylsuccinate belongs to the class of medicines called antibiotics, which are used to treat a variety of bacterial infections. Erythromycin ethylsuccinate is prescribed for infections of the middle ear and respiratory tract, because it prevents the bacteria from growing.

Erythromycin ethylsuccinate is effective only against bacterial infections, not those caused by viruses, parasites, or yeast.

Usual Dose

Infants and Children: 30–50 mg/kg/day divided into equal doses given every 6–8 hours. Maximum dose 2 g/day.

Adults: 400–800 mg/dose given every 6–12 hours.

Medication Interactions

Erythromycin ethylsuccinate may increase the risk for the development of adverse side effects of:

astemizole	methylprednisolone
carbamazepine	terfenadine
digoxin	theophylline
loratadine	warfarin

Adverse Side Effects

Minor: Nausea, vomiting, diarrhea, upset stomach, sore mouth, fatigue, darkened tongue.

Severe: Rash, fever, hives, stomach pain or cramps, hearing loss, yellow skin or eyes.

Storage and Administration

The oral medicine should be stored in a cool, dry place away from light. Prolonged exposure to heat, moisture, or light can damage the medicine.

Brand Names

E.E.S. 200
(liquid)

E.E.S. 400
(film-coated
tablet, liquid)

E.E.S. Granules
(liquid)

EryPed
(chewable
tablet, liquid)

EryPed 200
(liquid)

EryPed 400
(liquid)

Before the dose is measured, the liquid form of this medicine should be shaken well. Refrigeration of the liquid is recommended to preserve its taste. After receiving the liquid medicine from the pharmacy, it is good only for 14 days; therefore, always check the expiration date on the prescription label before using.

If the liquid comes in a dropper bottle, double check the instructions on the label. Some oral solutions come in dropper bottles, and may cause harm if applied to the eye or ear.

If upset stomach occurs, the medicine can be given with food or milk.

The film-coated tablet should be swallowed whole with a full glass of water. Do not crush or allow the child to chew it.

The chewable tablet should be chewed thoroughly before it is swallowed.

Special Instructions

The child's physician should be notified if the infection worsens or does not improve within 3–5 days.

N o t e s

Erythromycin stearate

Common Uses

Erythromycin stearate belongs to the class of medicines called antibiotics, which are used to treat a variety of bacterial infections. Erythromycin stearate is prescribed for infections of the middle ear and respiratory tract, because it prevents the bacteria from growing.

Erythromycin stearate is effective only against bacterial infections, not those caused by viruses, parasites, or yeast.

Usual Dose

Infants and Children: 20–40 mg/kg/day divided into equal doses given every 6 hours. Maximum dose 2 g/day.

Adults: 250–500 mg/dose given every 6–12 hours.

Medication Interactions

Erythromycin stearate may increase the risk for the development of adverse side effects of:

astemizole	methylprednisolone
carbamazepine	terfenadine
digoxin	theophylline
loratadine	warfarin

Adverse Side Effects

Minor: Nausea, vomiting, diarrhea, upset stomach, sore mouth, fatigue, darkened tongue.

Severe: Rash, fever, hives, stomach pain or cramps, hearing loss, yellow skin or eyes.

Storage and Administration

The oral medicine should be stored in a cool, dry place away from light. Prolonged exposure to heat, moisture, or light can damage the medicine.

Brand Names

Eramycin
(tablet)
Erythrocin
Stearate
(tablet)

E

Should be taken on an empty stomach (1 hour before a meal or 2–3 hours after a meal).

The tablet should be taken with a full glass of water.

If the child is unable to swallow the nonchewable tablet, it can be crushed and mixed with water or soft food (such as applesauce, pudding, jam, or jelly). This mixture should be swallowed and not chewed. The entire mixture must be swallowed to ensure that the child received the entire dose.

Do not allow the child to drink fruit juice 1 hour before or 1 one hour after taking erythromycin stearate.

Special Instructions

The child's physician should be notified if the infection worsens or does not improve within 3–5 days.

N o t e s

Erythromycin with Sulfisoxazole

Common Uses

Erythromycin with sulfisoxazole is a combination medicine that belongs to the class of medicines called antibiotics. This combination contains 200 mg of erythromycin and 600 mg of sulfisoxazole. Antibiotics are used to treat a variety of bacterial infections. Erythromycin with sulfisoxazole is pre-scribed for infections of the respiratory tract and middle ear, because it prevents the bacteria from growing.

Erythromycin with sulfisoxazole is effective only against bacterial infections, not those caused by viruses, parasites, or yeast.

Usual Dose

Children 2 months and older: 40–50 mg/kg/day of erythromycin and 150 mg/kg/day of sulfisoxazole divided into equal doses given every 6–8 hours. Maximum dose 2 g/day of erythromycin and 6 g/day of sulfisoxazole.

Adults: 400 mg of erythromycin and 1200 mg of sulfisoxazole given every 6 hours.

Medication Interactions

Erythromycin with sulfisoxazole may increase the risk for the development of adverse side effects of:

acetohexamide	methylprednisolone
astemizole	terfenadine
carbamazepine	theophylline
chlorpropamide	tolazamide
digoxin	tolbutamide
glipizide	warfarin
loratadine	

Brand Names

Eryzol
  (liquid)
Pediazole
  (liquid)

E

Adverse Side Effects

Minor: Nausea, vomiting, diarrhea, upset stomach, sore mouth, fatigue, darkened tongue, headache, increased sensitivity to sunlight, dizziness.

Severe: Rash; fever; hives; stomach pain or cramps; hearing loss; yellow skin or eyes; aching joints or muscles; numbness, tingling, or burning in the feet or hands; blood in the urine; painful urination; difficulty swallowing; low back pain; neck swelling; unusual bruising or bleeding.

Storage and Administration

Before the dose is measured, the liquid form of erythromycin with sulfisoxazole should be shaken well. Refrigeration of the liquid is recommended. After receiving the liquid medicine from the pharmacy, it is good only for 14 days; therefore, always check the expiration date on the prescription label before using.

Have the child take this medicine with a full glass of water and drink plenty of water in between doses.

If upset stomach occurs, the medicine can be given with food.

Special Instructions

The child's physician should be notified if the infection worsens or does not improve within 3–5 days.

This medication may make the child more sensitive to sunlight, so until it is known how he will respond, avoid prolonged exposure to the sun.

May cause dizziness in some people. Until it is known how the child will react to the medicine, activities that require mental alertness (such as physical education and playground activity) should be restricted.

N o t e s

Ethambutol E

Common Uses

Ethambutol belongs to the class of medicines called antituberculars. Ethambutol is prescribed for tuberculosis, because it prevents the bacteria from growing.

Ethambutol is effective only against tuberculosis, not infections caused by other bacteria, viruses, parasites, or yeast.

Brand Name

Myambutol (tablet)

Usual Dose

Children: 15 mg/kg/dose given once a day.

Adolescents and Adults: 15–25 mg/kg/dose given once a day or 50 mg/kg/dose twice a week. Maximum dose 2.5 g/day.

Medication Interactions

No major medication interactions have been found with other oral medications.

Adverse Side Effects

Minor: Nausea, vomiting, upset stomach, headache, dizziness.

Severe: Blurred vision, red–green color blindness, fever, sore throat, hallucinations, fatigue, rash, joint pain, numbness or tingling in the hands or feet, unusual bruising or bleeding, yellow skin or eyes.

Storage and Administration

The oral medicine should be stored in a cool, dry place away from light. Prolonged exposure to heat, moisture, or light can damage the medicine.

If upset stomach occurs, ethambutol can be given with food.

If the child is unable to swallow the tablet, it can be crushed and mixed with a small amount of water or soft food (such as applesauce, pudding, jam, or jelly). This mixture should be swallowed and not chewed. The entire mixture must be swallowed to ensure that the child received the full dose.

E

Special Instructions

Report any changes in the child's vision to her physician immediately.

May cause sedation, drowsiness, and dizziness in some people. Until it is known how the child will react to the medicine, activities that require mental alertness (such as physical education and playground activity) should be restricted.

N o t e s

Ethosuximide

E

Common Uses

Ethosuximide belongs to the class of medicines called anticonvulsants. Ethosuximide is used to treat and control seizures, because it alters the activity of chemicals in the brain that are responsible for the seizure.

Usual Dose

Children 3–6 years old: 15–40 mg/kg/day divided into equal doses given twice a day.

Children older than 6 years and Adults: 20–40 mg/kg/day divided into equal doses given twice a day.

Medication Interactions

No major medication interactions have been found with other oral medications.

Adverse Side Effects

Minor: Nausea, diarrhea, constipation, upset stomach, hiccups, drowsiness, dizziness, headache, skin rash.

Severe: Blurred vision, sore throat, fever, unusual bruising or bleeding, confusion, joint pain, loss of coordination, blood in the urine, depression, eye or tongue swelling.

Storage and Administration

The oral medicine should be stored in a cool, dry place away from light. Prolonged exposure to heat, moisture, or light can damage the medicine.

The liquid may be stored at room temperature and does not need to be refrigerated.

If upset stomach occurs, the medicine can be given with food or milk.

Brand Name

Zarontin
 (capsule,
 liquid)

E

If the child is unable to swallow the capsule, it can be opened and mixed with soft food (such as applesauce, pudding, jam, or jelly). This mixture should be swallowed and not chewed. The entire mixture must be swallowed to ensure that the child received the full dose.

Special Instructions

May cause sedation, drowsiness, and dizziness in some people. Until it is known how the child will react to the medicine, activities that require mental alertness (such as physical education and playground activity) should be restricted.

Do not suddenly stop giving ethosuximide to the child unless instructed to do so by a physician. Suddenly stopping this medication may cause severe seizures to occur.

Notes

Felbamate F

Common Uses

Felbamate belongs to the class of medicines called anticonvulsants. Felbamate is used to treat and control seizures; its mechanism of action is undetermined. However, it is thought that felbamate works by preventing the spread of the seizure and/or increasing the difficulty for a seizure to occur.

Brand Name

Felbatol
(tablet, liquid)

Usual Dose

Children 2–14 years old: Start with 15 mg/kg/day divided into equal doses given 3–4 times a day. Gradually increase the dose according to the physician's directions to 45 mg/kg/day.

Children older than 14 years and Adults: Start with 1200 mg/day divided into equal doses given 3–4 times a day. Gradually increase the dose according to the physician's directions to as high as 3600 mg/day if needed to control the seizures.

Medication Interactions

Medications that may decrease the effectiveness of felbamate are:

carbamazepine

phenytoin

Felbamate may increase the risk for the development of adverse side effects of:

phenytoin

Felbamate may decrease the effectiveness of:

carbamazepine

Adverse Side Effects

Minor: Nausea, vomiting, diarrhea, upset stomach, constipation, dizziness, drowsiness, dry mouth, nervousness, trembling, increased sensitivity to sunlight.

F

Severe: Stomach pain, confusion, fever, chills, sore throat, chest pain, changes in vision, hallucinations, unusual bruising or bleeding, yellow skin or eyes.

Storage and Administration

The oral medicine should be stored in a cool, dry place away from light. Prolonged exposure to heat, moisture, or light can damage the medicine.

Before the dose is measured, the liquid form of felbamate should be shaken well. The liquid may be stored at room temperature and does not need to be refrigerated.

If upset stomach occurs, the medicine can be given with food.

Special Instructions

May cause sedation, drowsiness, and dizziness in some people. Until it is known how the child will react to the medicine, activities that require mental alertness (such as physical education and playground activity) should be restricted.

Have the child avoid prolonged exposure to sunlight because this medication causes him to be more sensitive to it.

Do not suddenly stop giving felbamate to the child unless instructed to do so by a physician. Suddenly stopping this medication may cause severe seizures to occur.

For older children, dry mouth may be relieved by chewing gum or sucking on hard candy or ice chips. Younger children may need extra liquids.

N o t e s

Ferrous gluconate

Common Uses

Ferrous gluconate belongs to the class of medicines called iron salts. Ferrous gluconate is used to treat and prevent anemia caused by low amounts of iron in the body.

Usual Dose*

TREATMENT

Children: 3–6 mg of iron/kg/day divided into equal doses given 1–3 times a day.

Adults

TABLET, CAPSULE, LIQUID: 60 mg of iron/dose given 2–4 times a day.

LONG-ACTING TABLET: 50 mg of iron/dose given 1–2 times a day.

PREVENTION

Children: 1–2 mg of iron/kg/dose given once a day.

Adults: 60 mg of iron/dose given once a day.

*1 mg of iron = 8.3 mg of ferrous gluconate

Medication Interactions

A medication that may increase the risk for the development of ferrous gluconate adverse side effects is:

chloramphenicol

A medication that may decrease the effectiveness of ferrous gluconate is:

antacids

Ferrous gluconate may decrease the effectiveness of:

ciprofloxacin	minocycline
demeclocycline	norfloxacin
doxycycline	ofloxacin
enoxacin	oxytetracycline
lomefloxacin	penicillamine
methacycline	tetracycline

Brand Names

Fergon
 (tablet, liquid)
Ferralet
 (tablet)
Ferralet Slow
 Release
 (long-acting
 tablet)
Simron
 (capsule)

F

Adverse Side Effects

Minor: Nausea, vomiting, upset stomach, diarrhea, constipation, drowsiness, fatigue, black stools.

Severe: Chest pain; fast heartbeat; heartburn; blue lips, hands, or fingernail beds; pale or sweaty skin; throat pain; difficult or painful swallowing; stomach cramps or pain; blood in stool; seizures; unusual fatigue or weakness.

Storage and Administration

The oral medicine should be stored in a cool, dry place away from light. Prolonged exposure to heat, moisture, or light can damage the medicine.

Ferrous gluconate works best when taken on an empty stomach (1 hour before a meal or 2–3 hours after a meal). However, if upset stomach occurs it can be given with food or milk.

If the child is unable to swallow pills, the tablet can be crushed or the capsule opened and mixed with at least a half glass of water or juice or a small amount of soft food (such as applesauce, pudding, jam, or jelly). This mixture should be swallowed and not chewed. The entire mixture must be swallowed to ensure that the child received the full dose.

The long-acting tablet should be swallowed whole with a full glass of water. Do not crush it or allow the child to chew it.

Mix the liquid medicine with at least one-half a glass of water or juice and have the child drink the mixture through a straw. Do not allow the child to drink directly from the glass because ferrous gluconate may temporarily darken the teeth.

Do not allow the child to take antacids; drink milk, tea, or coffee; or eat cheese, yogurt, or eggs within 2 hours before or 2 hours after taking ferrous gluconate.

Special Instructions

May cause drowsiness in some people. Until it is known how the child will react to the medicine, activities that require mental alertness (such as physical education and playground activity) should be restricted.

May cause the stool to become black in color. This effect is harmless. If the black stool is tarry looking or has blood in it; or stomach cramps, pain, or discomfort occur, contact the child's physician.

Ferrous sulfate F

Common Uses

Ferrous sulfate belongs to the class of medicines called iron salts. Ferrous sulfate is used to treat and prevent anemia caused by low amounts of iron in the body.

Usual Dose

TREATMENT

Children: 3–6 mg of iron/kg/day divided into equal doses given 1–3 times a day.

Adults

TABLET, CAPSULE, LIQUID: 60 mg of iron/dose given 2–4 times a day.

LONG-ACTING TABLET: 50 mg of iron/dose given 1–2 times a day.

PREVENTION

Children: 1–2 mg of iron/kg/dose given once a day.

Adults: 60 mg of iron/dose given once a day.

Medication Interactions

A medication that may increase the risk for the development of ferrous sulfate adverse side effects is:

chloramphenicol

A medication that may decrease the effectiveness of ferrous sulfate is:

antacids

Ferrous sulfate may decrease the effectiveness of:

ciprofloxacin	minocycline
demeclocycline	norfloxacin
doxycycline	ofloxacin
enoxacin	oxytetracycline
lomefloxacin	penicillamine
methacycline	tetracycline

Brand Names

Feosol
(tablet,[a]
long-acting
capsule,[a]
liquid[b])

Feratab
(tablet[b])

Fer-In-Sol
(capsule,[a]
liquid[b])

Fero-Gradumet
Filmtab
(long-acting
tablet[b])

Ferospace
(capsule[b])

Ferralyn
Lanacaps
(long-acting
capsule[b])

Ferra-TD
(long-acting
capsule[b])

Mol-Iron
(tablet[b])

Slow FE
(long-acting
tablet[a])

[a]1 mg of iron =
3.1 mg of
Ferrous sulfate
[b]1 mg of iron =
5 mg of
Ferrous sulfate

F

Adverse Side Effects

Minor: Nausea, vomiting, upset stomach, diarrhea, constipation, drowsiness, fatigue, black stools.

Severe: Fast heartbeat; heartburn; blue lips, hands, or fingernail beds; pale or sweaty skin; difficult or painful swallowing; stomach cramps; blood in stool.

Storage and Administration

The oral medicine should be stored in a cool, dry place away from light. Prolonged exposure to heat, moisture, or light can damage the medicine.

Ferrous sulfate works best when taken on an empty stomach (1 hour before a meal or 2–3 hours after a meal). However, if upset stomach occurs it can be given with food or milk.

If the child is unable to swallow pills, the tablet can be crushed or the capsule opened and mixed with at least one-half a glass of water or juice or a small amount of soft food (such as applesauce, pudding, jam, or jelly). This mixture should be swallowed and not chewed. The entire mixture must be swallowed to ensure that the child received the full dose.

The long-acting tablet and long-acting capsule should be swallowed whole with a full glass of water. Do not crush it or allow the child to chew it.

Do not allow the child to take antacids; drink milk, tea, or coffee; or eat cheese, yogurt, or eggs wtihin 2 hours before or 2 hours after taking ferrous sulfate.

Mix the liquid medicine with at least one-half a glass of water or juice and have the child drink the mixture through a straw. Do not allow the child to drink directly from the glass because ferrous sulfate may temporarily darken the teeth.

If the liquid medicine is going to be given directly from the dropper bottle without dilution, place the correct amount of drops on the back of the child's tongue and wash it down with water or juice.

If the liquid comes in a dropper bottle, double-check the instructions on the label. Some oral solutions come in dropper bottles, and may cause harm if applied to the eye or ear.

Special Instructions

May cause drowsiness in some people. Until it is known how the child will react to the medicine, activities that require mental alertness (such as physical education and playground activity) should be restricted.

May cause the stool to become black in color. This effect is harmless. If the black stool is tarry looking or has blood in it; or stomach cramps, pain, or discomfort occur, contact the child's physician.

Fluconazole F

Common Uses

Fluconazole belongs to the class of medicines called antifungals, which are used to treat infections caused by yeast (fungus). Fluconazole is prescribed for infections of the mouth, esophagus (eating tube), blood, and brain, because it prevents the yeast from growing and making the infection worse.

Fluconazole is effective only against yeast infections, not those caused by bacteria, viruses, or parasites.

Usual Dose

Children 3–13 years old: 3–6 mg/kg/dose given once a day has been used, but the effectiveness of no particular dose has been well established.

Adults

MOUTH AND ESOPHAGUS INFECTIONS: 200 mg/dose given once a day the first day; then, 100 mg/dose given once a day thereafter.

BLOOD AND BRAIN INFECTIONS: 400 mg/dose given once a day the first day; then, 200–400 mg/dose given once a day thereafter.

Medication Interactions

Fluconazole may increase the risk for the development of adverse side effects of:

astemizole

phenytoin

terfenadine

Adverse Side Effects

Minor: Nausea, vomiting, diarrhea, headache.

Severe: Stomach pain, loss of appetite, rash, itching, dark urine, yellow skin or eyes.

Brand Name

Diflucan
(tablet, liquid)

F

Storage and Administration

The oral medicine should be stored in a cool, dry place away from light. Prolonged exposure to heat, moisture, or light can damage the medicine.

Before the dose is measured, the liquid form of fluconazole should be shaken well. The liquid may be stored at room temperature and does not need to be refrigerated. After receiving the liquid medicine from the pharmacy, it is good only for 14 days; therefore, always check the expiration date on the prescription label before using.

Fluconazole works best when taken on an empty stomach (1 hour before a meal or 2–3 hours after a meal), but if upset stomach occurs it can be given with food or milk.

If the child is unable to swallow the tablet, it can be crushed and mixed with water or soft food (such as applesauce, pudding, jam, or jelly). This mixture should be swallowed and not chewed. The entire mixture must be swallowed to ensure that the child received the full dose.

Special Instructions

The child's physician should be notified if the infection worsens or does not improve within 1–2 weeks.

N o t e s

Flunisolide

Common Uses

Flunisolide belongs to the class of medicines called corticosteroids. Oral inhalation of the medicine is used to prevent asthma attacks. Nasal inhalation is used to provide relief of stuffy nose, nasal irritation, and discomfort due to hay fever and allergies. Flunisolide is effective because it affects many different substances in the body that may cause or worsen these conditions.

Usual Dose

ORAL INHALATION

See the Medication Administration section for instructions on the proper use of an oral inhaler (page 10).

Children 4–15 years old: 1–2 inhalations 2 times a day. Maximum dose 4 inhalations/day.

Children older than 15 years and Adults: 2 inhalations 2 times a day. Maximum dose 8 inhalations/day.

NASAL INHALATION

See Medication Administration section for instructions on the proper use of a nasal inhaler (page 16).

Children 6–14 years old: 1 spray in each nostril 2–3 times a day or 2 sprays in each nostril 2 times a day. Maximum dose 4 sprays in each nostril/day.

Children older than 14 years and Adults: 2 sprays in each nostril 2 times a day. Maximum dose 8 sprays in each nostril/day

Medication Interactions

No major medication interactions have been found with other oral medications.

Adverse Side Effects

Minor

ORAL INHALATION: Yeast growth in mouth, hoarseness, dry mouth, bad taste in the mouth, cough, headache, dizziness.

Brand Names

AeroBid
(oral inhaler)
AeroBid M
(oral inhaler)
Nasalide
(nasal inhaler)

NASAL INHALATION: Irritation and burning of the nose, sneezing, yeast growth in the nose, headache, stuffy or runny nose, bad taste in the mouth, dizziness.

Severe: Rash, difficulty swallowing, hives, increased thirst.

Storage and Administration

The inhaler should be kept in a cool place. Do not puncture or expose the inhaler to prolonged periods of heat.

For proper use of the oral and nasal inhalers read the appropriate medication administration section.

If the child is also taking an orally inhaled bronchodilator (such as albuterol, metaproterenol, or terbutaline) give the entire bronchodilator dose at least 10–15 minutes, or as directed by a physician, before giving flunisolide oral inhalations.

After oral inhalation, have the child gargle or rinse his mouth with water. This helps prevent some of the side effects associated with oral inhalation.

Special Instructions

Oral inhalation of flunisolide is used to prevent asthma attacks, but it can not treat an asthma attack. When an asthma attack occurs this medicine will not help.

May cause dizziness in some people. Until it is known how the child will react to the medicine, activities that require mental alertness (such as physical education and playground activity) should be restricted.

N o t e s

Fluoxetine hydrochloride

Common Uses

Fluoxetine belongs to the class of medicines called antidepressants. Fluoxetine is used to treat various forms of depression, because it increases the concentration of a chemical in the brain that helps counteract the depression.

Usual Dose

Children 6–17 years old: 20 mg/day divided into equal doses given 1–2 times a day has been used, but the effectiveness of no particular dose has been well established.

Adults: 20 mg/day divided into equal doses given 1–2 times a day. Maximum dose 80 mg/day.

Medication Interactions

Fluoxetine may increase the risk for the development of adverse side effects of:

amitriptyline	doxepin
carbamazepine	imipramine
desipramine	nortriptyline

Adverse Side Effects

Minor: Nausea, vomiting, upset stomach, diarrhea, constipation, dizziness, drowsiness, agitation, nervousness, insomnia, decreased ability to concentrate, trembling, increased or decreased appetite, weight loss or gain, headache, increased sweating, flushing of skin, vision changes, changes in taste, dry mouth, fast heartbeat, frequent urination.

Severe: Anxiety, fever, chills, seizures, difficulty breathing, chest pain, rash, itchy skin, joint or muscle pain, swelling of the legs or feet, swelling of armpits or area under jaw, blurred vision, stomach pain.

Brand Name

Prozac
(capsule,
liquid)

Storage and Administration

The oral medicine should be stored in a cool, dry place away from light. Prolonged exposure to heat, moisture, or light can damage the medicine.

The liquid may be stored at room temperature and does not need to be refrigerated.

It is best to take fluoxetine with food to decrease or prevent upset stomach.

If the child is unable to swallow the capsule, it can be opened and mixed with water, apple juice, orange juice, or soft food (such as applesauce, pudding, jam, or jelly). This mixture should be swallowed and not chewed. The entire mixture must be swallowed to ensure that the child received the full dose.

Special Instructions

May cause drowsiness or dizziness in some people. Until it is known how the child will react to the medicine, activities that require mental alertness (such as physical education and playground activity) should be restricted.

For older children, dry mouth may be relieved by chewing gum or sucking on hard candy or ice chips. Younger children may need extra liquids

Do not allow the child to abruptly stop taking fluoxetine. Suddenly stopping the medicine can cause nausea, headache, or upset stomach.

N o t e s

Furosemide

F

Common Uses

Furosemide belongs to the class of medicines called diuretics. Furosemide is used to treat hypertension and remove excess body fluid caused by certain diseases because it increases the volume of urine removed from the body.

Usual Dose

Infants and Children: 1–2 mg/kg/dose given every 6–12 hours. Maximum dose 6 mg/kg/day.

Adults: 20–80 mg/day divided into equal doses given 1–2 times a day. Maximum dose 600 mg/day.

Medication Interactions

Medications that may increase the risk for the development of furosemide adverse side effects are:

chlorothiazide

hydrochlorothiazide

Furosemide may increase the risk for the development of adverse side effects of:

chlorothiazide

digoxin

hydrochlorothiazide

Adverse Side Effects

Minor: Blurred vision, constipation, diarrhea, upset stomach, headache, sore mouth, increased sensitivity to sunlight.

Severe: Muscle cramps or weakness, vomiting, confusion, weak pulse, abnormal heart rate, awareness of heartbeat, difficulty breathing, dry mouth, joint pain or swelling, mood changes, sore throat, tingling in fingers or toes, yellow skin or eyes, unusual bruising or bleeding, fatigue, fainting, ringing in the ears, fever, excessive thirst, low blood pressure, side or stomach pain, rash.

Brand Name

Lasix
(tablet,
liquid)

F

Storage and Administration

The oral medicine should be stored in a cool, dry place away from light. Prolonged exposure to heat, moisture, or light can damage the medicine.

The liquid may be stored at room temperature and does not need to be refrigerated.

If upset stomach occurs, the medicine can be given with food or milk.

If the child is unable to swallow the furosemide tablet, it can be crushed and mixed with water or soft food (such as applesauce, pudding, jam, or jelly). This mixture should be swallowed and not chewed. The entire mixture must be swallowed to ensure that the child received the full dose.

Special Instructions

May cause dizziness in some people. Until it is known how the child will react to the medicine, activities that require mental alertness (such as physical education and playground activity) should be restricted.

May cause dizziness upon standing; therefore, always have the child stand up slowly. If the child becomes dizzy, he should be instructed to sit or lie down immediately.

Have the child avoid prolonged exposure to sunlight, because furosemide causes him to be more sensitive to it.

N o t e s

Gabapentin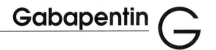

Common Uses

Gabapentin belongs to the class of medicines called anticonvulsants. Gabapentin treats and controls seizures by an undetermined mechanism. It is thought that gabapentin works by binding to an area of the brain to prevent a seizure from occurring or spreading.

Usual Dose

Children older than 12 years and Adults: 900–1800 mg/day divided into equal doses and given 3 times a day. Doses up to 3600 mg/day have been used.

Medication Interactions

A medication that may decrease the effectiveness of gabapentin is:

antacids

Adverse Side Effects

Minor: Nausea, vomiting, dizziness, drowsiness, fatigue, weight gain, dry mouth or throat.

Severe: Difficulty breathing, drooping eyelids, trembling, double vision, slurred speech, diarrhea, severe sedation or drowsiness, tiredness or fatigue, decreased mental awareness, irregular heartbeat, blood in stools, stomach pain, unusual bruising or bleeding, personality change, agitation, aggressive behavior.

Storage and Administration

The oral medicine should be stored in a cool, dry place away from light. Prolonged exposure to heat, moisture, or light can damage the medicine.

If upset stomach occurs, the medicine can be given with food.

Brand Name

Neurontin
(capsule)

If the child is unable to swallow the capsule, it can be opened and mixed with a small amount of water, fruit juice, or soft food (such as applesauce, pudding, jam, or jelly). This mixture should be swallowed and not chewed. The entire mixture must be swallowed to ensure that the child received the full dose.

Do not allow the child to take antacids within 2 hours before or 2 hours after taking gabapentin.

Special Instructions

May cause drowsiness or dizziness in some people. Until it is known how the child will react to the medicine, activities that require mental alertness (such as physical education and playground activity) should be restricted.

For older children, dry mouth may be relieved by chewing gum or sucking on hard candy or ice chips. Younger children may need extra liquids.

Do not suddenly stop giving gabapentin to the child unless instructed to do so by a physician. Suddenly stopping this medication may cause severe seizures to occur.

N o t e s

Guaifenesin G

Common Uses

Guaifenesin belongs to the class of medicines called expectorants. Guaifenesin is used to relieve and control coughs due to the common cold, because it helps increase the removal of mucus from the chest.

Usual Dose

Children younger than 2 years: 12 mg/kg/day divided into equal doses given 6 times a day.

Children 2–5 years old: 50–100 mg/dose given every 4 hours. Maximum dose 600 mg/day.

Children 6–12 years old: 100–200 mg/dose given every 4 hours. Maximum dose 1200 mg/day.

Children older than 12 years and Adults: 200–400 mg/dose given every 4 hours. Maximum dose 2400 mg/day.

Medication Interactions

No major medication interactions have been found with other oral medications.

Adverse Side Effects

Minor: Drowsiness, nausea, diarrhea.

Severe: Vomiting, stomach pain, rash, headache, fever.

Storage and Administration

The oral medicine should be stored in a cool, dry place away from light. Prolonged exposure to heat, moisture, or light can damage the medicine.

The liquid may be stored at room temperature and does not need to be refrigerated.

Guaifenesin should be given with a full glass of water and the child should drink plenty of water between doses.

Brand Names

Anti-Tuss
(liquid)

Glyate
(liquid)

Guiatuss
(liquid)

Halotussin
(liquid)

Humibid L.A.
(long-acting
tablet)

Humibid
Sprinkle
(long-acting
capsule)

Hytuss
(tablet)

Hytuss 2X
(capsule)

Mytussin
(liquid)

Robitussin
(liquid)

Scot-tussin
Expectorant
(liquid)

Uni-tussin
(liquid)

The long-acting tablet should be swallowed whole with a full glass of water. Do not crush or allow the child to chew it.

If the child is unable to swallow pills, the non–long-acting tablets can be crushed or the capsules (long-acting and non–long-acting) can be opened and mixed with soft food (such as applesauce, pudding, jam, or jelly). This mixture should be swallowed and not chewed. The entire mixture must be swallowed to ensure that the child received the full dose.

Special Instructions

May cause drowsiness in some people. Until it is known how the child will react to the medicine, activities that require mental alertness (such as physical education and playground activity) should be restricted.

N o t e s

Haloperidol

Common Uses

Haloperidol belongs to the class of medicines called tranquilizers. Haloperidol is used to treat various forms of mental illness and agitation, because it blocks a chemical that is responsible for imbalanced nerve transmissions in the brain.

Brand Name

Haldol
(tablet,
concentrate)

Usual Dose

Children 3–12 years old or 15–40 kg (33–88 lb): 0.01–0.03 mg/kg/day divided into equal doses and given 1–3 times a day. Maximum dose 0.15 mg/kg/day.

Children older than 12 years and Adults: 0.5–5 mg/dose given 2–3 times a day. Maximum dose 30 mg/day.

Medication Interactions

Medications that may decrease the effectiveness of haloperidol are:

atropine   oxybutynin

benztropine   scopolamine

carbamazepine   trihexyphenidyl

A medication that may cause weakness; lethargy; trembling; confusion; stupor; fever; rigidity or immobility; restlessness and agitation; involuntary movements of the face, mouth, and tongue; or dystonia (muscle spasms, difficulty with speech or swallowing) when combined with haloperidol is:

lithium

Adverse Side Effects

Minor: Dry mouth, constipation, dizziness, drowsiness, stuffy nose, restlessness, pink or red-brown urine, increased sensitivity to sunlight.

Severe: Chest pain; seizures; difficulty swallowing or breathing; fever; sore throat; rash; stomach pain; yellow skin or eyes; unusual bruising or bleeding; blurred vision; trembling; twitching; drooling; unintentional movements of the face, mouth, and tongue.

Storage and Administration

The oral medicine should be stored in a cool, dry place away from light. Prolonged exposure to heat, moisture, or light can damage the medicine.

The concentrate may be stored at room temperature and does not need to be refrigerated.

Keep the haloperidol concentrate out of sunlight because this will damage the medicine.

Haloperidol works best when taken on an empty stomach (1 hour before a meal or 2–3 hours after a meal), but if upset stomach occurs it can be given with food or milk.

Avoid touching the concentrate or having it touch the child's skin because an itchy rash may occur.

The concentrate should be mixed with half a cup or more of apple juice, orange juice, water, carbonated beverage, or a small amount of soft food (such as applesauce, pudding, jam, or jelly). Prepare the mixture just before giving the dose. The medicine will be damaged if left in the mixture; therefore, do not premix and store.

If the child is unable to swallow the tablet, it can be crushed and mixed with water or juice. The entire mixture must be swallowed to ensure that the child received the full dose.

Special Instructions

May cause drowsiness and dizziness in some people. Until it is known how the child will react to the medicine, activities that require mental alertness (such as physical education and playground activity) should be restricted.

May cause dizziness upon standing; therefore, always have the child stand up slowly. If the child becomes dizzy, he should be instructed to sit or lie down immediately.

Limit the child's playing on hot days, because the medicine increases the risk of heat stroke.

For older children, dry mouth may be relieved by chewing gum or sucking on hard candy or ice chips. Younger children may need extra liquids.

May cause the urine to become pink to red-brown in color. This effect is harmless.

Have the child avoid prolonged exposure to sunlight, because haloperidol may cause him to be more sensitive to it.

N o t e s

Hydralazine hydrochloride

Common Uses

Hydralazine belongs to the class of medicines called vasodilators. Hydralazine is used to treat and control high blood pressure and weak hearts, because it dilates the blood vessels, allowing blood to move through the vessels more easily.

Usual Dose

Children: 0.75–3 mg/kg/day divided into equal doses given every 6–12 hours. Increase the dose according to the physician's directions until the desired effect is obtained. Maximum dose 7.5 mg/kg/day or 200 mg/day.

Adults: 10–50 mg/dose given four times a day. Increase the dose according to the physician's directions until the desired effect is obtained. Maximum dose 300 mg/day.

Medication Interactions

Medications that may increase the risk for the development of hydralazine adverse side effects are:

metoprolol

propranolol

Hydralazine may increase the risk for the development of adverse side effects of:

metoprolol

propranolol

zalcitabine

Adverse Side Effects

Minor: Constipation, diarrhea, nausea, vomiting, headache, dizziness, drowsiness, flushing, loss of appetite, nasal congestion, watery eyes.

Severe: Chest pain, confusion, cramping, painful or difficult urination, fever, sore throat, itching, numbness or tingling in fingers or toes, awareness of heartbeat, fast heartbeat, rash, difficulty breathing, unusual bruising or bleeding, yellow skin or eyes, prolonged fatigue, aching muscles or joints, sudden weight gain (3–5 lb), swelling of the legs or feet.

Storage and Administration

The oral medicine should be stored in a cool, dry place away from light. Prolonged exposure to heat, moisture, or light can damage the medicine.

Hydralazine works best when given with food or milk to increase the amount of medicine that the body absorbs and to prevent upset stomach.

If the child is unable to swallow the tablet, it can be crushed and mixed with water or soft food (such as applesauce, pudding, jam, or jelly). This mixture should be swallowed and not chewed. The entire mixture must be swallowed to ensure that the child received the full dose.

Special Instructions

May cause drowsiness or dizziness in some people. Until it is known how the child will react to the medicine, activities that require mental alertness (such as physical education and playground activity) should be restricted.

May cause dizziness upon standing; therefore, always have the child stand up slowly. If she becomes dizzy, she should be instructed to sit or lie down immediately.

N o t e s

Hydrochlorothiazide

Brand Names

Esidrix
(tablet)
HydroDIURIL
(tablet)
Hydro-Par
(tablet)
Oretic
(tablet)

Generic
medicine
dosage form:
Hydrochloro-
thiazide
(tablet, liquid)

Common Uses

Hydrochlorothiazide belongs to the class of medicines called diuretics. Hydrochlorothiazide treats hypertension and removes excess body fluid caused by certain diseases by increasing the volume of urine removed from the body.

Usual Dose

Children younger than 6 months: 2–3.3 mg/kg/day divided into equal doses given 2 times a day.

Children 6 months–2 years old: 12.5–37.5 mg/day divided into equal doses given 2 times a day.

Children 2–12 years old: 37.5–100 mg/day divided into equal doses given 2 times a day.

Children older than 12 years and Adults: 25–100 mg/day divided into equal doses given 1–2 times a day. Maximum dose 200 mg/day.

Medication Interactions

Medications that may increase the risk for the development of hydrochlorothiazide adverse side effects are:

bumetanide

ethacrynic acid

furosemide

Medications that may decrease the effectiveness of hydrochlorothiazide are:

cholestyramine

colestipol

Hydrochlorothiazide may increase the risk for the development of adverse side effects of:

bumetanide	ethacrynic acid
diazoxide	furosemide
digoxin	lithium

Hydrochlorothiazide may decrease the effectiveness of:

acetohexamide	glyburide
chlorpropamide	tolazamide
glipizide	tolbutamide

Adverse Side Effects

Minor: Constipation, diarrhea, upset stomach, cramps, dizziness, drowsiness, headache, restlessness, increased sensitivity to sunlight.

Severe: Muscle cramps or weakness, vomiting, confusion, weak pulse, abnormal heart rate, awareness of heartbeat, difficulty breathing, dry mouth, swollen or painful joints, mood changes, sore throat, tingling in fingers or toes, yellow skin or eyes, unusual bruising or bleeding, fever, excessive thirst, itching, rash, low blood pressure.

Storage and Administration

The oral medicine should be stored in a cool, dry place away from light. Prolonged exposure to heat, moisture, or light can damage the medicine.

The liquid may be stored at room temperature and does not need to be refrigerated.

If upset stomach occurs, the medicine can be given with food or milk.

If the child is unable to swallow the hydrochlorothiazide tablet, it can be crushed and mixed with water or soft food (such as applesauce, pudding, jam, or jelly). This mixture should be swallowed and not chewed. The entire mixture must be swallowed to ensure that the child received the full dose.

Special Instructions

May cause dizziness and drowsiness in some people. Until it is known how the child will react to the medicine, activities that require mental alertness (such as physical education and playground activity) should be restricted.

May cause dizziness upon standing; therefore, always have the child stand up slowly. If the child becomes dizzy, he should be instructed to sit or lie down immediately.

Have the child avoid prolonged exposure to sunlight, because this medication causes him to be more sensitive to it.

H ydrocortisone

Brand Names

Aeroseb-HC
(skin aerosol)
Ala-Cort
(skin lotion)
Ala-Scalp
(skin lotion)
Anusol-HC 2.5%
(skin cream)
Bactine
Hydrocortisone
(skin cream)
Cetacort
(skin lotion)
CortaGel
(skin gel)
Cortaid
(skin aerosol)
Cort-Dome
(skin cream,
rectal
suppository)
Cortef
(tablet, liquid)
Cortizone•5
(skin ointment,
skin cream)

(continued next page)

Common Uses

Hydrocortisone belongs to the class of medicines called corticosteroids. Oral tablets and liquids are used to treat inflammatory diseases and various other problems. Skin creams, lotions, ointments, gels, and skin aerosols are used to relieve the itching, redness, and discomfort of various skin diseases and rashes caused by poison oak and poison ivy. Rectal creams, ointments, and suppositories are used to relieve the itching and discomfort of various problems of the rectum. Hydrocortisone is effective because it affects many different substances in the body that may cause or worsen these conditions.

Usual Dose

TABLET AND LIQUID

Children: 2.5–10 mg/kg/day divided into equal doses given every 6–8 hours.

Adults: 20–240 mg/day divided into equal doses given every 6–12 hours.

SKIN OINTMENT, CREAM, GEL, LOTION, AND AEROSOL:

Children and Adults: Apply as directed to the affected area 2–4 times a day.

RECTAL SUPPOSITORY AND CREAM:

Children and Adults: 1 applicator full of cream or ointment or 1 suppository inserted 1–2 times a day.

Medication Interactions

A medication that may increase the risk for the development of hydrocortisone adverse side effects is:

troleandomycin

Medications that may decrease the effectiveness of hydrocortisone are:

phenobarbital

phenytoin

primidone

rifampin

Hydrocortisone decreases the effectiveness of:

aspirin	phenytoin
bismuth subsalicylate	salsalate
choline salicylate	sodium salicylate
magnesium salicylate	

Adverse Side Effects

Minor

TABLET AND LIQUID: Round face, weight gain, acne, upset stomach, nausea, vomiting, increased appetite, dizziness.

SKIN PREPARATIONS: Acne, dry skin, mild burning or stinging sensation, itching, minor rash.

RECTAL PREPARATIONS: Muscle weakness, round face, weight gain, acne, upset stomach, nausea, vomiting.

Severe: Rash; hives; skin blistering; loss of skin color; skin infection at the site where the medicine is used; difficulty swallowing; increased thirst; headache; seizures; insomnia; fatigue; abnormal hair growth; dizziness; black, tarry stools; sore throat; fever; hallucinations; irregular heartbeat; blurred vision; stomach pain; nightmares; difficulty breathing; unusual weakness; leg cramps.

Brand Names

(continued)

Cortizone•10
(skin ointment)

Dermolate
(skin cream)

1% HC
(skin ointment)

Hycort
(skin ointment, skin cream)

HydroTex
(skin cream)

Hytone
(skin ointment, skin cream, skin lotion)

Nutracort
(skin lotion)

Proctocort
(rectal cream)

Synacort
(skin cream)

Tegrin-HC
(skin ointment)

H

Storage and Administration

Before the dose is measured, the liquid form of hydrocortisone should be shaken well. The liquid may be stored at room temperature and does not need to be refrigerated.

The oral medicine should be stored in a cool, dry place away from light. Prolonged exposure to heat, moisture, or light can damage the medicine.

The skin preparations may be stored at room temperature.

The rectal suppository and cream may be stored at room temperature.

If the child is unable to swallow the tablet, it can be crushed and mixed with a small amount of water or soft food (such as applesauce, pudding, jam, or jelly). This mixture should be swallowed and not chewed. The entire mixture must be swallowed to ensure that the child received the full dose.

It is best to have the child take this medicine with food or milk to decrease or prevent stomach upset.

Special Instructions

May cause dizziness in some people. Until it is known how the child will react to the medicine, activities that require mental alertness (such as physical education and playground activity) should be restricted.

Skin medicine is to be used only on the skin; be careful not to get it into the child's eyes.

Do not use tight-fitting diapers when the skin medicine is being applied to the diaper area.

The child's physician should be notified if black, tarry stools occur.

If the child has been taking hydrocortisone for more than 1 week, do not abruptly stop it. Suddenly stopping the oral medicine (tablet or liquid) can cause nausea, vomiting, weakness, fever, shortness of breath, stomach or back pain, or dizziness.

If the child has been taking this medicine for more than 1 week, notify the child's physician if a serious injury or illness occurs.

Ibuprofen

Common Uses

Ibuprofen belongs to the class of medicines called nonsteroidal antiinflammatory drugs (NSAIDs). Ibuprofen is used to relieve fever and mild-to-moderate pain, because it blocks the production of chemicals that cause pain and inflammation.

Usual Dose

FEVER

Children 6 months–12 years old: 5–10 mg/kg/dose given every 6–8 hours. Maximum dose 40 mg/kg/day.

Children older than 12 years and Adults: 200–400 mg/dose given every 4–6 hours. Maximum dose 1200 mg/day.

PAIN RELIEF (NON-ARTHRITIS PAIN)

Children: 4–10 mg/kg/dose given every 6–8 hours.

Adults: 200–400 mg/dose given every 4–6 hours. Maximum dose 1200 mg/day.

ARTHRITIS PAIN

Children: 30–50 mg/kg/day divided into equal doses given every 6 hours. Maximum dose 2400 mg/day.

Children who weigh more than 40 kg (88 lb) and Adults: 400–800 mg/dose given every 6–8 hours. Maximum dose 3200 mg/day.

Medication Interactions

Ibuprofen may increase the risk for the development of adverse side effects of:

lithium

Brand Names

Advil
(tablet)

Excedrin IB
(tablet)

Ibuprin
(tablet)

Medipren
(tablet)

Midol 200
(tablet)

Motrin IB
(tablet)

Nuprin
(tablet)

Pamprin-IB
(tablet)

PediaProfen
(liquid)

I

Ibuprofen may decrease the effectiveness of:

acebutolol	metoprolol
atenolol	nadolol
bumetanide	pindolol
ethacrynic acid	propranolol
furosemide	timolol

Adverse Side Effects

Minor: Nausea, vomiting, diarrhea, constipation, upset stomach, bloating, drowsiness, sweating, nervousness, dizziness, headache, depression, insomnia.

Severe: Black or tarry stools, difficulty breathing, increased sensitivity to sunlight, blurred vision, ringing or buzzing in ears, stomach pain, seizures, confusion, awareness of heartbeat, fast heartbeat, rash, unusual bruising or bleeding, yellow skin or eyes, unexplained weakness or fatigue, unusual weight gain, sore throat, fever, chills, persistent headache, difficult urination, green urine, blood in the urine, eye pain.

Storage and Administration

The oral medicine should be stored in a cool, dry place away from light. Prolonged exposure to heat, moisture, or light can damage the medicine.

Before the dose is measured, the liquid form of ibuprofen should be shaken well. The liquid may be stored at room temperature and does not need to be refrigerated.

Ibuprofen works best when taken on an empty stomach (1 hour before a meal or 2–3 hours after a meal), but if upset stomach occurs it can be given with food or milk.

This medicine should be taken with a full glass of water.

If the child is unable to swallow the ibuprofen tablet, it can be crushed and mixed with water or soft food (such as applesauce, pudding, jam, or jelly). This mixture should be swallowed and not chewed. The entire mixture must be swallowed to ensure that the child received the full dose.

Special Instructions

May cause dizziness or drowsiness in some people. Until it is known how the child will react to the medicine, activities that require mental alertness (such as physical education and playground activity) should be restricted.

Have the child avoid prolonged exposure to sunlight because this medication may cause him to be more sensitive to it.

The child's physician should be notified at once if there is blood in the urine or black, tarry stools.

N o t e s

mipramine hydrochloride

Brand Names

Janimine
(tablet)
Tofranil
(tablet)
Tofranil-PM
(capsule)

Common Uses

Imipramine belongs to the class of medicines called tricyclic antidepressants. Imipramine is used to treat people with various forms of depression, because it increases the concentration of chemicals in the brain that help counteract the depression. Imipramine also can be used to treat certain types of nerve pain, and in children, it can be used to treat bed-wetting.

Usual Dose

Start with the lowest dose and increase it according to the physician's directions.

DEPRESSION

Children: 1.5–5 mg/kg/day divided into equal doses given 1–4 times a day.

Adolescents: 25–100 mg/day divided into equal doses given as a single or divided dose.

Adults: 75–300 mg/day divided into equal doses given 1–4 times a day.

BED-WETTING

Children 6 years and older: Start with 10–25 mg/dose given at bedtime. Increase the dose according to the physician's directions. Maximum dose 6–12 years: 50 mg/dose; 13 years and older: 75 mg/dose

Medication Interactions

Medications that increase the risk for the development of imipramine adverse side effects are:

cimetidine

fluoxetine

Imipramine decreases the effectiveness of:

clonidine

guanethidine

Imipramine increases the risk for the development of bleeding when given with:

dicumarol

Medications that may cause seizures, dangerous increases in body temperature, or death when combined with imipramine are:

isocarboxazid

phenelzine

tranylcypromine

Adverse Side Effects

Minor: Sedation, drowsiness, dry mouth, bad taste in the mouth, constipation, fatigue, insomnia, dizziness, increased sensitivity to sunlight, nervousness, anxiety, sweating, nausea, vomiting.

Severe: Blurred vision, confusion; seizures; chest pain; fever; sore throat; hallucinations; irregular heartbeat; stomach pain; loss of balance; unusual bruising or bleeding; yellow skin or eyes; joint pain; swollen breasts; trembling; unintentional movements of the face, mouth, and tongue.

Storage and Administration

The oral medicine should be stored in a cool, dry place away from light. Prolonged exposure to heat, moisture, or light can damage the medicine.

Imipramine works best when taken on an empty stomach (1 hour before a meal or 2–3 hours after a meal), but if upset stomach occurs it can be given with food or milk.

If the child is unable to swallow pills, the tablet can be crushed or the capsules opened and mixed with a small amount of water or soft food (such as applesauce, pudding, jam, or jelly). This mixture should be swallowed and not chewed. The entire mixture must be swallowed to ensure that the child received the full dose.

Special Instructions

May cause sedation, drowsiness, and dizziness in some people. Until it is known how the child will react to the medicine, activities that require mental alertness (such as physical education and playground activity) should be restricted.

May cause dizziness upon standing; therefore, always have the child stand up slowly. If the child becomes dizzy, she should be instructed to sit or lie down immediately.

Have the child avoid prolonged exposure to sunlight, because this medication may cause her to be more sensitive to it.

For older children, dry mouth may be relieved by chewing gum or sucking on hard candy or ice chips. Younger children may need extra liquids.

In children with a seizure disorder, this medicine may cause seizures even if the child's condition is currently controlled.

N o t e s

Indomethacin

Common Uses

Indomethacin belongs to the class of medicines called nonsteroidal antiinflammatory drugs (NSAIDs). Indomethacin is used to relieve mild-to-moderate pain because it blocks the production of chemicals that cause pain and inflammation.

Usual Dose

Children: 1–2 mg/kg/day divided into equal doses given 2–4 times a day. Maximum dose 4 mg/kg/day or 200 mg/day.

Adults: 25–50 mg/dose given 2–4 times a day. Maximum dose 200 mg/day. The long-acting capsule should be taken only 1–2 times a day.

Medication Interactions

Indomethacin may increase the risk for the development of adverse side effects of:

digoxin

lithium

Indomethacin may decrease the effectiveness of:

acebutolol	lisinopril
atenolol	metoprolol
benazepril	nadolol
bumetanide	pindolol
captopril	propranolol
enalapril	quinapril
ethacrynic acid	ramipril
fosinopril	timolol
furosemide	

Brand Names

Indocin (capsule, liquid)

Indocin SR (long-acting capsule)

Indomethacin SR (long-acting capsule)

Adverse Side Effects

Minor: Nausea, vomiting, diarrhea, constipation, upset stomach, bloating, drowsiness, nervousness, sweating, dizziness, headache, depression, insomnia.

Severe: Black or tarry stools, difficulty breathing, increased sensitivity to sunlight, blurred vision, ringing or buzzing in ears, stomach pain, seizures, confusion, awareness of heartbeat, fast heartbeat, rash, unusual bruising or bleeding, yellow skin or eyes, unexplained weakness or fatigue, unusual weight gain, sore throat, fever, chills, persistent headache, difficult urination, green urine, blood in the urine, eye pain.

Storage and Administration

The oral medicine should be stored in a cool, dry place away from light. Prolonged exposure to heat, moisture, or light can damage the medicine.

Before the dose is measured, the liquid form of indomethacin should be shaken well. The liquid may be stored at room temperature and does not need to be refrigerated.

It is best to give this medicine with food or milk to decrease or prevent upset stomach.

The long-acting capsule should be swallowed whole with a full glass of water. Do not crush or allow the child to chew it.

If the child is unable to swallow the non–long-acting capsule, it can be opened and mixed with soft food (such as applesauce, pudding, jam, or jelly). This mixture should be swallowed and not chewed. The entire mixture must be swallowed to ensure that the child received the full dose.

Special Instructions

May cause drowsiness and dizziness in some people. Until it is known how the child will react to the medicine, activities that require mental alertness (such as physical education and playground activity) should be restricted.

Have the child avoid prolonged exposure to sunlight because this medication may cause him to be more sensitive to it.

The child's physician should be notified at once if there is blood in the urine or black, tarry stools.

Insulin

Common Uses

Insulin belongs to the class of medicines called anti-diabetics. Insulin is used to treat diabetes that can not be controlled by pills or diet, because it replaces naturally occurring insulin when not enough is being produced by the body.

Usual Dose

Children and Adults: 0.5–1.0 units/kg/day divided into doses given 1–4 times a day. The dose is adjusted according to the physician's directions until the desired effect is obtained.

Adolescents (during growth spurt): 0.8–1.2 units/kg/day divided into doses given 1–4 times a day. The dose is adjusted according to the physician's directions until the desired effect is obtained.

Medication Interactions

Medications that may increase the risk for the development of low blood sugar when combined with insulin are:

alcohol	magnesium salicylate
aspirin	pargyline
bismuth subsalicylate	phenelzine
choline salicylate	salsalate
clofibrate	sodium salicylate
isocarboxazid	tranylcypromine

Medications that may hide the symptoms of low blood sugar when combined with insulin are:

carteolol	pindolol
nadolol	propranolol
penbutolol	timolol

See the Medication Administration section for instructions on the proper way to give insulin injections (page 17).

Brand Names

Humulin 70/30 (solution for injection)

Humulin L (solution for injection)

Humulin N (solution for injection)

Humulin R (solution for injection)

Lente Insulin (solution for injection)

Novolin 70/30 (solution for injection)

Novolin L (solution for injection)

Novolin N (solution for injection)

Novolin R (solution for injection)

NPH Insulin (solution for injection)

Regular Insulin (solution for injection)

Ultralente U (solution for injection)

Velosulin Human (solution for injection)

Adverse Side Effects

Minor: Redness, itching, stinging, or swelling at site of the injection.

Severe: Symptoms of low blood sugar (see Special Instructions), difficulty breathing.

Storage and Administration

The medicine should be stored in a cool place away from light. Prolonged exposure to heat or light can damage the medicine.

Opened vials can be kept at room temperature for 1 month. Unopened vial should be kept refrigerated until opened.

Before measuring the dose, roll the insulin vial between your hands to mix the medicine. Do not shake the vial.

Mix different types of insulin only when directed by the physician. If mixing is necessary, regular insulin (signified by the word "regular" or the letter "R") should be measured in the syringe first before the other insulin is measured.

Frequently changing the site of insulin injection is recommended to avoid problems associated with multiple single-site injections.

Always measure the dose immediately prior to giving the insulin. Never premeasure and store the medicine.

Special Instructions

Always observe the child for the following symptoms: unusual fatigue, drowsiness, headache, dizziness, sweating, trembling, nervousness, unusual hunger, nausea, fast heartbeat, tingling of fingers, muscle weakness, blurred vision, fainting, chills, restlessness, cold sweats. If any of these symptoms occur the child may be experiencing hypoglycemia (low blood sugar). If a blood monitoring device is present, measure the child's blood sugar and record it for the physician. Have the child drink a glass of orange juice or eat a candy bar, honey, or a sugar cube. Watch the child closely and call his physician.

Isoniazid

Common Uses

Isoniazid belongs to the class of medicines called anti-tuberculars, which are used to treat tuberculosis and prevent its occurrence. Isoniazid is prescribed for this infection because it prevents the bacteria from growing.

Isoniazid is not effective against infections caused by other bacteria, viruses, parasites, or yeast.

Brand Names

Laniazid
(tablet)
Laniazid C.T.
(tablet)

Generic
medicine
dosage form:
Isoniazid
(tablet, liquid)

Usual Dose

TREATMENT

Infants and Children

10–20 mg/kg/day divided into equal doses given 1–2 times a day. Maximum dose 300 mg/day.

or

20–40 mg/kg/dose given twice a week. Maximum dose 900 mg/dose.

Adults

5 mg/kg/dose given once a day. Maximum dose 300 mg/day.

or

15 mg/kg/dose given twice a week. Maximum dose 900 mg/dose.

PREVENTION

Infants and Children: 10 mg/kg/dose given once a day. Maximum dose 300 mg/day.

Adults: 300 mg/dose given once a day.

Medication Interactions

Isoniazid may increase the risk for the development of adverse side effects of:

phenytoin

zalcitabine

Medications that may increase the risk for the development of liver toxicity when combined with isoniazid are:

carbamazepine

rifampin

Adverse Side Effects

Minor: Nausea, upset stomach, dizziness, heartburn, confusion, breast enlargement.

Severe: Blurred vision or other visual changes, eye pain, dark urine, fever, sore throat, rash, seizure, numbness, burning or tingling in the fingers or toes, unusual bruising or bleeding, fatigue, weakness, yellow skin or eyes, memory loss, muscle or joint pain, vomiting, swollen glands.

Storage and Administration

The oral medicine should be stored in a cool, dry place away from light. Prolonged exposure to heat, moisture, or light can damage the medicine.

The liquid may be stored at room temperature and does not need to be refrigerated.

Isoniazid works best when taken on an empty stomach (1 hour before a meal or 2–3 hours after a meal), but if upset stomach occurs it can be given with food or milk.

If the child is unable to swallow the tablet, it can be crushed and mixed with a small amount of water or soft food (such as applesauce, pudding, jam, or jelly). This mixture should be swallowed and not chewed. The entire mixture must be swallowed to ensure that the child received the full dose.

Special Instructions

May cause dizziness in some people. Until it is known how the child will react to the medicine, activities that require mental alertness (such as physical education and playground activity) should be restricted.

Ingestion of certain foods (smoked fish, skipjack, tuna, yeast extracts, sausages, sauerkraut juice, and several cheeses) may cause sweating, itching, headache, low or high blood pressure, and awareness of heartbeat. These foods should be avoided while taking this medicine.

In children with a seizure disorder, this medicine may cause seizures even if the child's condition is currently controlled.

N o t e s

K etoconazole

Common Uses

Ketoconazole belongs to the class of medicines called antifungals, which are used to treat infections caused by yeast (fungus). Ketoconazole is prescribed for infections of the mouth, esophagus (eating tube), blood, skin, and brain, because it prevents the yeast from growing.

Ketoconazole is effective only against yeast infections, not those caused by bacteria, viruses, or parasites.

Usual Dose

TABLET

Children older than 2 years: 5–10 mg/kg/day divided into equal doses given 1–2 times a day. Maximum dose 800 mg/day.

Adults: 200–400 mg/dose given once a day.

CREAM AND SHAMPOO

Children: No doses have been determined, but the adult doses may possibly be used.

Adults

CREAM: Apply as directed to the infected area 1–2 times a day.

SHAMPOO: Wash hair with the medicine 2 times a week.

Medication Interactions

Medications that may decrease the effectiveness of ketoconazole are:

antacids	nizatidine
cimetidine	ranitidine
famotidine	rifampin

Ketoconazole may increase the risk for the development of adverse side effects of:

astemizole   prednisolone

cyclosporine   prednisone

methylprednisolone   terfenadine

Ketoconazole may decrease the effectiveness of:

rifampin

Adverse Side Effects

Minor

TABLETS: Diarrhea, headache, insomnia, loss of appetite, dizziness, drowsiness, increased sensitivity to sunlight.

SKIN MEDICINE AND SHAMPOO: Dry skin, mild burning or stinging sensation, itching, mild redness of skin.

Severe: Severe diarrhea, stomach pain, fever, chills, rash, hives, skin blistering, severe skin irritation, scalp blisters, abnormal hair loss, dark urine, unusual fatigue, yellow skin or eyes.

Storage and Administration

The oral medicine should be stored in a cool, dry place away from light. Prolonged exposure to heat, moisture, or light can damage the medicine.

The skin cream and shampoo may be stored at room temperature.

It is best to give ketoconazole with food or milk to increase the amount of medicine the body absorbs and to help prevent upset stomach.

Do not allow the child to take antacids within 2 hours before or 2 hours after taking ketoconazole.

K

If the child is unable to swallow the ketoconazole tablet, it can be crushed and mixed with fruit juice or soft food (such as applesauce, pudding, jam, or jelly). This mixture should be swallowed and not chewed. The entire mixture must be swallowed to ensure that the child received the full dose.

Some children may have to take this medicine with dilute hydrochloric acid (HCl) to help the body absorb the medicine. If no other instructions on the proper preparation and administration are available, follow the directions below:

1. Dissolve the tablet in 4 ml of HCl provided by the pharmacy.

2. Add 1–2 teaspoons of water to this mixture.

3. Have the child sip the mixture through a straw that is placed as far back into her throat as possible. If this mixture touches her teeth, the HCl can damage them.

4. When the child has finished drinking the mixture, have her rinse her mouth with a half glass of water. The water should be swished around the entire mouth and then swallowed.

Apply shampoo to wet hair, then lather and wash the hair. Let the medicine stay in the hair for about 1 minute before rinsing. Reapply the medicine and rewash. Let the medicine stay in the hair for approximately 3 minutes, then rinse the hair.

Special Instructions

May cause drowsiness or dizziness in some children. Until it is known how the child will react to the medicine, activities that require mental alertness (such as physical education and playground activity) should be restricted.

Skin cream is to be used only on the skin; be careful not to get it into the child's eyes.

Have the child avoid prolonged exposure to sunlight, because this medication causes her to be more sensitive to it.

N o t e s

L evothyroxine sodium

Brand Names

Levothroid
(tablet)

Levoxine
(tablet)

Synthroid
(tablet)

Common Uses

Levothyroxine belongs to the class of medicines called thyroid hormones. Levothyroxine is used to replace the naturally occurring thyroid hormone when the thyroid gland can not produce enough.

Usual Dose

Children younger than 6 months: 8–10 mcg/kg/dose given once a day.

Children 6–12 months old: 6–8 mcg/kg/dose given once a day.

Children 1–5 years old: 5–6 mcg/kg/dose given once a day.

Children 6–12 years old: 4–5 mcg/kg/dose given once a day.

Children older than 12 years: 2–3 mcg/kg/dose given once a day.

Adults: 12.5–50 mcg/dose given once a day. Adjust the dose according to the physician's directions until the desired effect is obtained.

Medication Interactions

Medications that may decrease the effectiveness of levothyroxine are:

cholestyramine   iron salts

Levothyroxine may increase the risk for the development of adverse side effects of:*

dicumarol   warfarin

Levothyroxine may decrease the effectiveness of:*

digitoxin   theophylline

digoxin

*These interactions depend on how well the thyroid disease is controlled and if the medications were started before or after levothyroxine.

Adverse Side Effects

Minor: Constipation, dry skin, fatigue, weight gain.

Severe: Diarrhea, vomiting, rash, weight loss, sweating, insomnia, headache, trembling, nervousness, fever, intolerance to heat, leg cramps, muscle ache, difficulty breathing, chest pain, awareness of heartbeat, fast heartbeat.

Storage and Administration

The oral medicine should be stored in a cool, dry place away from light. Prolonged exposure to heat, moisture, or light can damage the medicine.

Levothyroxine works best when taken on an empty stomach (1 hour before a meal or 2–3 hours after a meal), but if upset stomach occurs it can be given with food.

If the child is unable to swallow the tablet, it can be crushed and mixed with a small amount of water or soft food (such as applesauce, pudding, jam, or jelly). This mixture should be swallowed and not chewed. The entire mixture must be swallowed to ensure that the child received the full dose.

Special Instructions

Always observe the child for the following symptoms: unusual fatigue or drowsiness, headache, weakness, intolerance to cold, decreased or increased sweating, muscle cramps or pain, constipation, diarrhea, difficulty breathing, swelling of arms or legs, slow heartbeat, awareness of heartbeat, pale skin, weight loss, intolerance to heat, trembling, irritability, and insomnia.

If any of the above symptoms occur the child may be receiving an incorrect dose of levothyroxine. Notify the child's physician so appropriate treatment can be started.

L indane

Brand Names

G-well
(skin lotion,
hair shampoo)
Kwell
(skin cream,
skin lotion,
hair shampoo)
Scabene
(hair
shampoo)

Common Uses

Lindane belongs to both the scabicides and pediculicides classes of medicines. Lindane is used to treat and prevent the spread of head lice, crabs, and scabies, because it kills the live lice, crabs, and scabies and their eggs.

Lindane treats only head lice, crabs, and scabies—not infections caused by bacteria, viruses, parasites, or yeasts.

Usual Dose

SCABIES

CREAM AND LOTION: Apply to the entire body, from the neck to the soles of the feet (for infants also apply to the head). Thoroughly remove the medicine with water after it has remained on the body for 6 hours for infants, 6–8 hours for children, and 8–12 hours for adults.

HEAD LICE AND CRABS

CREAM AND LOTION: Apply to the infected area, and allow it to remain there for 8–12 hours. Then remove with water.

SHAMPOO: Apply to dry hair and leave in place for approximately 4 minutes. Add small amounts of water until a lather develops, then scrub and rinse with water. Use a special comb that either comes with the medicine or can be purchased at the pharmacy to remove the eggs.

Medication Interactions

Medications that may increase the risk for developing seizures when combined with lindane are:

oil-based hair and skin products

Adverse Side Effects

Minor: Skin irritation or redness.

Severe: Seizures, dizziness, muscle cramps, awareness of heartbeat, nervousness, vomiting.

Storage and Administration

The skin cream, skin lotion, and hair shampoo should be stored in a cool, dry place away from light. Prolonged exposure to heat, moisture, or light can damage the medicine.

Before the dose is measured, the lotion form of lindane should be shaken well.

Lindane can be absorbed through the skin. Therefore, to avoid adverse side effects, wear gloves while applying the medicine.

Do not use lindane in areas where there are cuts or wounds.

One application usually is enough to cure the infection. If another application is necessary, wait 7 days before reapplying the medicine.

Special Instructions

Skin cream, lotion, and hair shampoo are to be used only on the skin and hair; be careful not to get the medication into the child's eyes.

Children and adults with a seizure disorder may be at an increased risk for developing seizures when using lindane.

To remove all lice, crabs, and scabies from bed linens, towels, and clothes, wash them in hot water or have them dry cleaned. Combs and brushes should be soaked in boiling water for 1 hour. This must be done the same day the medicine is applied to ensure that reinfection does not occur.

N o t e s

L oracarbef

Lorabid
(capsule,
liquid)

Common Uses

Loracarbef belongs to the class of medicines called antibiotics, which are used to treat a variety of bacterial infections. Loracarbef is prescribed for infections of the middle ear, respiratory tract, urinary tract, and skin, because it prevents the bacteria from growing.

Loracarbef is effective only against bacterial infections, not those caused by viruses, parasites, or yeast.

Usual Dose

Children 6 months–12 years old: 15–30 mg/kg/day divided into equal doses given every 12 hours.

Children older than 12 years and Adults: 200–400 mg/dose given every 12 hours or 200 mg/dose given every 24 hours.

Medication Interactions

No major medication interactions have been found with other oral medications.

Adverse Side Effects

Minor: Nausea, vomiting, diarrhea, dizziness, upset stomach, headache.

Severe: Rash, hives, difficulty breathing, seizures, severe diarrhea, unusual bruising or bleeding, stomach cramps, fatigue, joint pain, fever.

Storage and Administration

The oral medicine should be stored in a cool, dry place away from light. Prolonged exposure to heat, moisture, or light can damage the medicine.

Before the dose is measured, the liquid form of loracarbef should be shaken well. The liquid may be stored at room temperature and does not need to be refrigerated. After receiving the liquid medicine from the pharmacy, it is good only for 14 days; therefore, always check the expiration date on the prescription label before using.

Loracarbef works best when taken on an empty stomach (1 hour before a meal or 2–3 hours after a meal).

If the child is unable to swallow the capsule, it can be opened and mixed with a small amount of water or soft food (such as applesauce, pudding, jam, or jelly). This mixture should be swallowed and not chewed. The entire mixture must be swallowed to ensure that the child received the full dose.

Special Instructions

The child's physician should be notified if the infection worsens or does not improve within 3–5 days.

May cause dizziness in some people. Until it is known how the child will react to the medicine, activities that require mental alertness (such as physical education and playground activity) should be restricted.

N o t e s

M etaproterenol sulfate

Brand Names

Alupent
(tablet, liquid,
oral inhaler,
solution for
inhalation)

Metaprel
(tablet, liquid,
oral inhaler,
solution for
inhalation)

Common Uses

Metaproterenol belongs to the class of medicines called bronchodilators. Metaproterenol is used to treat and prevent asthma attacks and improve breathing difficulties caused by various other non–infection-related respiratory problems. Metaproterenol is able to treat these conditions because it opens the airways and prevents them from closing again.

Usual Dose

TABLET AND LIQUID

Children younger than 2 years: 0.4 mg/kg/dose given 3–4 times a day.

Children 2–6 years old: 1–2.6 mg/kg/day divided into equal doses given 3–4 times a day.

Children 6–9 years old: 10 mg/dose given 3–4 times a day.

Children older than 9 years and Adults: 20 mg/dose given 3–4 times a day.

ORAL INHALATION

See the Medication Administration section for instructions on the proper use of an oral inhaler (page 10).

Children older than 12 years and Adults: 2–3 puffs every 3–4 hours. Maximum dose 12 puffs/day.

SOLUTION FOR INHALATION

See the Medication Administration section for instructions on the proper use of a nebulizer (page 13).

Infants and Children: 0.01–0.02 ml/kg/dose of the 5% solution diluted in 2–3 ml of normal saline given every 4–6 hours.

Adolescents and Adults: 5–15 inhalations of the undiluted 5% solution given every 4–6 hours.

or

0.2–0.3 mL/dose of the 5% solution diluted with 2–3 mL of normal saline given every 4–6 hours.

Note: 0.2 mL of 5% solution = 2.5 ml of 0.4% solution.
0.3 mL of 5% solution = 2.5 mL of 0.6% solution.

Medication Interactions

No major medication interactions have been found with other oral medications.

Adverse Side Effects

Minor

ORAL INHALATION: Dry throat and mouth. Side effects listed under the Solution for Inhalation section also can occur if too many inhalations are given or if the medicine is given too often.

SOLUTION FOR INHALATION: Dry throat and mouth, nervousness, headache, fast heartbeat, trembling, dizziness, flushing.

TABLET AND SYRUP: Nervousness, headache, fast heartbeat, trembling, insomnia, increased blood pressure, dizziness, upset stomach, nausea, vomiting, hyperactivity, flushing.

Severe: Chest pain, hallucinations, difficult or painful urination, rash, irregular heartbeat.

Storage and Administration

The oral medicine should be stored in a cool, dry place away from light. Prolonged exposure to heat, moisture, or light can damage the medicine.

The metaproterenol liquid may be stored at room temperature and does not need to be refrigerated.

The inhaler should be kept in a cool place. Do not puncture or expose the inhaler to prolonged periods of heat.

The solution for inhalation should be stored in a cool, dry place away from light. Prolonged exposure to heat, moisture, or light can damage the medicine.

If upset stomach occurs, metaproterenol can be given with food.

For proper use of the oral inhaler and nebulizer read the appropriate medication administration sections.

M

To prevent dry throat and mouth, have the child rinse his mouth with water after each inhalation.

If the child is receiving more than 1 puff of the oral inhaler, give the second puff at least 1 minute after the first one.

If the child is receiving another inhaled medicine for asthma, the entire inhaled metaproterenol dose should be given at least 10–15 minutes before the other inhaled medicine is given, or as directed by a physician.

The tablet should be swallowed whole with a full glass of water. Do not crush or allow the child to chew it.

Special Instructions

Consult the child's physician about giving extra inhalations, because increasing the number of inhalations may be dangerous.

Children may be more susceptible to the side effects of insomnia, nervousness, hyperactivity, and fast heartbeat than adults.

Have the child avoid beverages containing caffeine and excessive amounts of chocolate because this may make the child susceptible to insomnia, irritability, and hyperactivity.

May cause dizziness in some children. Until it is known how the child will react to the medicine, activities that require mental alertness (such as physical education and playground activity) should be restricted.

For older children, dry mouth may be relieved by chewing gum or sucking on hard candy or ice chips. Younger children may need extra liquids.

N o t e s

Methylphenidate hydrochloride

Common Uses

Methylphenidate belongs to the class of medicines called stimulants, which are used to treat narcolepsy and attention deficit disorder with hyperactivity (ADDH). Methylphenidate is able to treat these conditions because it causes chemicals to be released into the brain, which allows more focused attention.

Usual Dose

NARCOLEPSY

Adults: 10 mg/dose given 2–3 times a day. Maximum dose 60 mg/day.

ATTENTION DEFICIT DISORDER WITH HYPERACTIVITY

Children older than 6 years: Start with 0.3 mg/kg/dose divided into equal doses or 2.5–5 mg/dose given before breakfast and lunch. Adjust the dose according to the physician's directions until the desired effect is obtained. Maximum dose 2 mg/kg/day or 60 mg/day.

Medication Interactions

Medications that increase the risk for the development of methylphenidate adverse side effects are:

furazolidone	sodium bicarbonate
potassium citrate	sodium citrate
sodium acetate	sodium lactate

Methylphenidate decreases the effectiveness of:

guanethidine

Medications that may cause dangerous increases in body temperature, brain hemorrhage, seizures, or even death when combined with methylphenidate are:

isocarboxazid	phenelzine
pargyline	tranylcypromine

Brand Names

Ritalin
  (tablet)
Ritalin-SR
  (long-acting
  tablet)

M

Adverse Side Effects

Minor: Upset stomach, nausea, dizziness, drowsiness, fatigue, dry mouth, headache, insomnia,
nervousness, loss of appetite.

Severe: Chest pain, fever, sore throat, hives, rash, hallucinations, joint pain, awareness of heartbeat, fast heartbeat, seizures, uncontrolled movements, unusual bruising or bleeding, blurred vision.

Storage and Administration

The oral medicine should be stored in a cool, dry place away from light. Prolonged exposure to heat, moisture, or light can damage the medicine.

It is best to give methylphenidate with food or milk to decrease or prevent upset stomach.

The long-acting tablet should be swallowed whole with a full glass of water. Do not crush or allow the child to chew it.

If the child is unable to swallow the non–long-acting tablet, it can be crushed and mixed with water, juice, or soft food (such as applesauce, pudding, jam, or jelly). The entire mixture must be swallowed to ensure that the child received the full dose.

Special Instructions

May cause drowsiness and dizziness in some people. Until it is known how the child will react to the medicine, activities that require mental alertness (such as physical education and playground activity) should be restricted.

For older children, dry mouth may be relieved by chewing gum or sucking on hard candy or ice chips. Younger children may need extra liquids.

Have the child avoid beverages containing caffeine, because this may make her susceptible to insomnia, irritability, and hyperactivity.

In children with a seizure disorder, this medicine may cause seizures even if the child's condition is currently controlled.

Eating certain foods while taking methylphenidate (cheese, avocado, bananas, homemade bread, canned meats, salami, sausage, pepperoni, liver, certain fish, pickled herring, bologna, marmite, soy sauce, chocolate, figs, raisins, and alcohol) may cause a dangerous increase in blood pressure. Check with the child's physician for a complete list of foods that should be avoided.

Metoclopramide M

Common Uses

Metoclopramide belongs to both the antivomiting and gastrointestinal (GI) stimulant medicine classes. Metoclopramide prevents nausea and vomiting by blocking impulses in the brain associated with these conditions. This medicine can also treat conditions when the airway is damaged by stomach acid (gastroesophageal reflux) and when the stomach fails to move (GI motility disorders), because it increases the ability of the stomach to empty its contents into the small intestine.

Usual Dose

VOMITING

Children and Adults: 1–2 mg/kg/dose given every 2–4 hours.

GASTROESOPHAGEAL REFLUX AND GI MOTILITY DISORDERS

Infants and Children: 0.2–0.4 mg/kg/day divided into equal doses given 4 times a day. Maximum dose 0.5 mg/kg/day.

Adults: 10–15 mg/dose given 4 times a day.

Medication Interactions

Metoclopramide may increase the risk for the development of adverse side effects of:

cyclosporine

Metoclopramide may decrease the effectiveness of:

digoxin

Adverse Side Effects

Minor: Nausea, diarrhea, constipation, dizziness, headache, insomnia, restlessness, drowsiness, fatigue.

Severe: Rash; wheezing; difficulty breathing; uncontrolled movements of face, eyes, arms, or legs; trembling; anxiety; confusion.

Brand Name

Reglan
(tablet, liquid)

M

Storage and Administration

The oral medicine should be stored in a cool, dry place away from light. Prolonged exposure to heat, moisture, or light can damage the medicine.

The liquid may be stored at room temperature and does not need to be refrigerated.

Metoclopramide should be taken 30 minutes before a meal and at bedtime.

If the child is unable to swallow the tablet, it can be crushed and mixed with a small amount of water or soft food (such as applesauce, pudding, jam, or jelly). This mixture should be swallowed and not chewed. The entire mixture must be swallowed to ensure that the child received the full dose.

Special Instructions

May cause drowsiness and dizziness in some children. Until it is known how the child will react to the medicine, activities that require mental alertness (such as physical education and playground activity) should be restricted.

For older children, dry mouth may be relieved by chewing gum or sucking on hard candy or ice chips. Younger children may need extra liquids.

N o t e s

Metronidazole M

Common Uses

Metronidazole belongs to the class of medicines called antibiotics, which are used to treat a variety of bacterial infections. Metronidazole is prescribed for infections of the skin and gut, because it prevents the bacteria from growing. Topically, metronidazole is used to treat acne.

Metronidazole is effective only against bacterial infections, not those caused by viruses, parasites, or yeast.

Usual Dose

TABLET

Children: 15–50 mg/kg/day divided into equal doses given every 6–8 hours. Maximum dose 2 g/day.

Adults: (Maximum dose 4 g/day.) 250–750 mg/dose given every 6–8 hours.

or

2 g as a single dose.

or

30 mg/kg/day divided into equal doses given every 6 hours.

SKIN GEL

Children: No dosage has been determined, but the adult doses may possibly be prescribed.

Adults: Apply as directed to the infected area twice a day.

Medication Interactions

Medications that may decrease the effectiveness of metronidazole are:

phenobarbital

primidone

Brand Names
Flagyl (tablet)
MetroGel (skin gel)
Protostat (tablet)

M

Metronidazole may increase the risk for the development of adverse side effects of:

warfarin

zalcitabine

A medication that may cause confusion and hallucinations when combined with metronidazole is:

disulfiram

A medication that may cause nausea, vomiting, red skin, awareness of heartbeat, and fast heartbeat when combined with metronidazole is:

alcohol

Adverse Side Effects

Minor

TABLET: Nausea, diarrhea, constipation, headache, metallic taste, dry mouth, dizziness, dark or reddish brown urine.

SKIN MEDICINE: Dry skin, mild burning or stinging sensation, itching, mild or temporary redness of skin.

Severe: Numbness or tingling in the hands or feet, furry tongue, seizures, hives, rash, skin blistering, severe skin irritation, joint pain, sore throat, fever.

Storage and Administration

The oral medicine should be stored in a cool, dry place away from light. Prolonged exposure to heat, moisture, or light can damage the medicine.

The skin gel may be stored at room temperature.

If upset stomach occurs, metronidazole can be given with food or milk.

If the child is unable to swallow the tablet, it can be crushed and mixed with water or soft food (such as applesauce, pudding, jam, or jelly). This mixture should be swallowed and not chewed. The entire mixture must be swallowed to ensure that the child received the full dose.

Special Instructions

The child's physician should be notified if the infection worsens or does not improve within 3–5 days.

May cause dizziness in some people. Until it is known how the child will react to the medicine, activities that require mental alertness (such as physical education and playground activity) should be restricted.

May cause the urine to become dark or reddish brown in color. This is a harmless side effect.

Skin gel is to be used only on the skin; be careful not to get it into the child's eyes.

In children with a seizure disorder, this medicine may cause seizures even if the child's condition is currently controlled.

For older children, dry mouth may be relieved by chewing gum or sucking on hard candy or ice chips. Younger children may need extra liquids.

Notes

M inocycline hydrochloride

Brand Name

Minocin
(capsule,
liquid)

Common Uses

Minocycline belongs to the class of medicines called antibiotics, which are used to treat a variety of bacterial infections. Minocycline is prescribed for infections of the genital and respiratory tract, and to prevent the spread of certain diseases. Minocycline is effective against these infections because it prevents the bacteria from growing.

Minocycline is effective only against bacterial infections, not those caused by viruses, parasites, or yeast.

Usual Dose

Children older than 8 years: 4 mg/kg, then 2 mg/kg/dose every 12 hours.

Adults: 200 mg, then 100 mg/dose given every 12 hours. Maximum dose 400 mg/day.

Medication Interactions

Medications that may decrease the effectiveness of minocycline are:

amoxicillin	penicillin G
ampicillin	penicillin V
antacids	potassium citrate
bismuth salts	sodium acetate
cloxacillin	sodium bicarbonate
dicloxacillin	sodium citrate
iron salts	sodium lactate
nafcillin	zinc gluconate
oxacillin	zinc sulfate

Minocycline increases the risk for the development of adverse side effects of:

digoxin

methoxyflurane

Adverse Side Effects

Minor: Diarrhea, nausea, upset stomach, dizziness, headache, increased sensitivity to sunlight, tooth discoloration in children who do not yet have permanent teeth.

Severe: Difficulty breathing, joint pain, rash, sore throat, fever, yellow skin or eyes, mouth irritation.

Storage and Administration

The oral medicine should be stored in a cool, dry place away from light. Prolonged exposure to heat, moisture, or light can damage the medicine.

Before the dose is measured, the liquid form of minocycline should be shaken well. The liquid may be stored at room temperature and does not need to be refrigerated.

Have the child take the capsules with a full glass of water.

If upset stomach occurs, minocycline can be given with food or milk.

Do not allow the child to take antacids within 2 hours before or 2 hours after taking minocycline.

If the child is unable to swallow the capsule, it can be opened and mixed with water or soft food (such as applesauce, pudding, jam, or jelly). This mixture should be swallowed and not chewed. The entire mixture must be swallowed to ensure that the child received the full dose.

Special Instructions

May cause dizziness in some people. Until it is known how the child will react to the medicine, activities that require mental alertness (such as physical education and playground activity) should be restricted.

The child's physician should be notified if the infection worsens or does not improve within 3–5 days.

Have the child avoid prolonged exposure to sunlight, because this medication causes him to be more sensitive to it.

Irreversible tooth discoloration may occur in the missing permanent teeth in children that do not have all their permanent teeth.

Nafcillin sodium

Brand Name

Unipen
(tablet,
capsule)

Common Uses

Nafcillin belongs to the class of medicines called antibiotics, which are used to treat a variety of bacterial infections. Nafcillin is prescribed for infections of the skin, soft tissue, respiratory tract, bone, and heart, because it prevents the bacteria from growing.

Nafcillin is effective only against bacterial infections, not those caused by viruses, parasites, or yeast.

Usual Dose

Children: 25–100 mg/kg/day divided into equal doses given every 6 hours.

Adults: 250–1000 mg/dose given every 4–6 hours.

Medication Interactions

Medications that decrease the effectiveness of nafcillin are:

demeclocycline   minocycline

doxycycline   oxytetracycline

methacycline   tetracycline

Adverse Side Effects

Minor: Diarrhea, nausea, vomiting, heartburn, upset stomach, darkened tongue.

Severe: Rash, hives, difficulty breathing, blood in the urine, sore throat, fever, stomach cramps, seizures, unexplained bleeding or bruising, severe diarrhea.

Storage and Administration

The oral medicine should be stored in a cool, dry place away from light. Prolonged exposure to heat, moisture, or light can damage the medicine.

Nafcillin works best when taken on an empty stomach (1 hour before a meal or 2–3 hours after a meal).

Special Instructions

The child's physician should be notified if the infection worsens or does not improve within 3–5 days.

N o t e s

N aproxen

Brand Names

Aleve
(tablet)
Anaprox
(tablet)
Anaprox DS
(tablet)
Naprosyn
(tablet, liquid)

Common Uses

Naproxen belongs to the class of medicines called nonsteroidal antiinflammatory drugs (NSAIDs). Naproxen is used to relieve mild-to-moderate pain because it blocks the production of chemicals that cause pain and inflammation.

Usual Dose

PAIN RELIEF (NON-ARTHRITIS)

Children older than 2 years: 5–7 mg/kg/dose given every 8–12 hours.

Adults: 500 mg the first dose, then 250 mg/dose given every 6–8 hours. Maximum dose 1250 mg/day.

ARTHRITIS PAIN

Children older than 2 years: 10–15 mg/kg/day divided into equal doses given twice a day.

Adults: 500–1000 mg/kg/day divided into equal doses given twice a day. Maximum dose 1500 mg/day.

Medication Interactions

Naproxen may increase the risk for the development of adverse side effects of:

lithium

Naproxen may decrease the effectiveness of:

acebutolol	nadolol
atenolol	penbutolol
betaxolol	pindolol
bisoprolol	propranolol
carteolol	sotalol
metoprolol	timolol

N

Adverse Side Effects

Minor: Dizziness, nausea, upset stomach, vomiting, headache, drowsiness, constipation, nervousness, sweating, acne.

Severe: Black or tarry stools, stomach pain, blurred vision, awareness of heartbeat, ringing in ears, rash, sore throat, fever, unusual bruising or bleeding, yellow skin or eyes, wheezing, difficulty breathing, blood in the urine, decreased hearing.

Storage and Administration

The oral medicine should be stored in a cool, dry place away from light. Prolonged exposure to heat, moisture, or light can damage the medicine.

Before the dose is measured, the liquid form of naproxen should be shaken well. The liquid may be stored at room temperature and does not need to be refrigerated.

Naproxen works best when taken on an empty stomach (1 hour before a meal or 2–3 hours after a meal), but if upset stomach occurs it can be given with food or milk.

Naproxen should be taken with a full glass of water.

If the child is unable to swallow the tablet, it can be crushed and mixed with water or soft food (such as applesauce, pudding, jam, or jelly). This mixture should be swallowed and not chewed. The entire mixture must be swallowed to ensure that the child received the full dose.

Special Instructions

May cause dizziness and drowsiness in some people. Until it is known how the child will react to the medicine, activities that require mental alertness (such as physical education and playground activity) should be restricted.

The child's physician should be notified at once if there is blood in the urine or black, tarry stools.

Have the child avoid prolonged exposure to sunlight, because this medication may cause her to be more sensitive to it.

N ifedipine

Brand Names

Adalat
(capsule)
Procardia
(capsule)
Procardia XL
(long-acting
tablet)

Common Uses

Nifedipine belongs to the class of medicines called calcium-channel blockers. Nifedipine is used to prevent the occurrence of chest pain and to treat and control high blood pressure, because it widens blood vessels of the heart and body and decreases the amount of oxygen needed by the heart.

Usual Dose

Children: 0.25–0.5 mg/kg/dose given every 6–8 hours. Maximum dose 180 mg/day.

Adults

CAPSULE: 10–30 mg/dose given every 6–8 hours. Maximum dose 180 mg/day.

LONG-ACTING TABLET: 30–60 mg/dose given every 24 hours. Maximum dose 120 mg/day.

Medication Interactions

A medication that may increase the risk for the development of nifedipine adverse side effects is:

cimetidine

Medications that may decrease the effectiveness of nifedipine are:

phenobarbital

primidone

Adverse Side Effects

Minor: Bloating, coughing, dizziness, flushing, headache, warm feeling, nasal congestion, nausea, sweating.

Severe: Blurred vision; chills; fever; rash; sore throat; confusion; difficulty breathing; fainting; mood changes; muscle cramps; trembling; slow heartbeat;

awareness of heartbeat; wheezing; swelling, tenderness, or easy bleeding of the gums.

Storage and Administration

The oral medicine should be stored in a cool, dry place away from light. Prolonged exposure to heat, moisture, or light can damage the medicine.

If upset stomach occurs, nifedipine can be given with food.

The capsule and long-acting tablet should be swallowed whole with a full glass of water. Do not crush or allow the child to chew it.

Special Instructions

May cause dizziness in some people. Until it is known how the child will react to the medicine, activities that require mental alertness (such as physical education and playground activity) should be restricted.

May cause dizziness upon standing; therefore, always have the child stand up slowly. If the child becomes dizzy, she should be instructed to sit or lie down immediately.

The empty long-acting tablet may be seen in the stool. This is normal and no extra doses need to be given.

The child may have a headache during the first few days of taking nifedipine. The headache may be relieved by taking the medicine with food. If the headache persists past the first few days, the child should be seen by her physician.

The child should brush and floss her teeth and massage the gums regularly and carefully. The dentist should be visited regularly.

N o t e s

N itrofurantoin

Brand Names

Furadantin
(liquid)

Furalan
(tablet)

Furanite
(tablet)

Macrodantin
(capsule)

Nitrofan
(capsule)

Common Uses

Nitrofurantoin belongs to the class of medicines called antibiotics, which are prescribed for a variety of bacterial infections. Nitrofurantoin is prescribed for infections of the urinary tract, and also prevent the return of a urinary tract infection, because it prevents the bacteria from growing.

Nitrofurantoin is effective only against bacterial infections, not those caused by viruses, parasites, or yeast.

Usual Dose

TREATMENT

Children: 5–7 mg/kg/day divided into equal doses given every 6 hours. Maximum dose 400 mg/day.

Adults: 50–100 mg/dose given every 6 hours.

PREVENTION

Children: 1–2 mg/kg/day divided into equal doses given every 12–24 hours. Maximum dose 400 mg/day.

Adults: 50–100 mg as a single dose given at bedtime.

Medication Interactions

Medications that may decrease the effectiveness of nitrofurantoin are:

magaldrate   magnesium hydroxide

magnesium carbonate   magnesium oxide

magnesium citrate   magnesium trisilicate

magnesium gluconate

Nitrofurantoin may increase the risk for the development of adverse side effects of:

zalcitabine

Adverse Side Effects

Minor: Headache, dizziness, drowsiness, paleness, tooth discoloration, upset stomach, dark yellow or brown urine.

Severe: Chest pain, hives, rash, difficulty breathing, chills, fever, fainting, irritation of the mouth, numbness or tingling of the hands or feet, yellow skin or eyes.

Storage and Administration

The oral medicine should be stored in a cool, dry place away from light. Prolonged exposure to heat, moisture, or light can damage the medicine.

Before the dose is measured, the liquid form of nitrofurantoin should be shaken well. The liquid may be stored at room temperature and does not need to be refrigerated.

It is best to give nitrofurantoin with food or milk to increase the amount of medicine taken into the body and to prevent upset stomach.

The tablets and capsules should be swallowed whole with a full glass of water. Do not crush, open, or allow the child to chew them because the contents may stain the teeth yellow.

The measured dose of the liquid form of nitrofurantoin should be diluted with milk, water, fruit juice, or infant formula to mask its bad taste. Have the child rinse his mouth after taking the medicine to prevent staining of the teeth.

Special Instructions

May cause dizziness and drowsiness in some people. Until it is known how the child will react to the medicine, activities that require mental alertness (such as physical education and playground activity) should be restricted.

The child's physician should be notified if the infection worsens or does not improve within 3–5 days.

May cause the urine to become dark yellow or brown in color. This effect is harmless.

N ystatin

Brand Names

Mycostatin
(tablet, liquid,
skin ointment,
skin cream,
skin powder)

Mycostatin
Pastilles
(lozenge)

Nilstat
(tablet, liquid,
oral powder,
skin ointment,
skin cream)

Nystex
(liquid,
skin ointment,
skin cream)

Common Uses

Nystatin belongs to the class of medicines called antifungals, which are used to treat infections caused by yeast (fungus). Nystatin can be used to treat infections of the mouth and skin, because it prevents the yeast from growing.

Nystatin is effective only against yeast infections, not those caused by bacteria, viruses, or parasites.

Usual Dose

LIQUID

Infants: 200,000 units/dose (2 mL) given 4 times a day, or 100,000 units (1 mL) applied with dropper to each side of the mouth 4 times a day.

Children and Adults: 400,000–600,000 units/dose (4–6 mL) given 4 times a day.

LOZENGE

Children and Adults: Dissolve 200,000–400,000 units/dose (1–2 lozenges) slowly in the mouth 4–5 times a day.

ORAL POWDER

Children and Adults: One-eighth of a teaspoon (500,000 units) mixed in one-half cup of water given 4 times a day.

TABLET

Adults: 500,000–1,000,000 units/dose given 3 times a day.

SKIN OINTMENT, CREAM, AND POWDER

Children and Adults: Apply as directed to the infected area 2–4 times a day.

Medication Interactions

No major medication interactions have been found with other oral medications.

Adverse Side Effects

Minor

ORAL MEDICINE: (usually seen with high doses) Diarrhea, upset stomach, nausea, vomiting.

SKIN MEDICINE: Dry skin, mild burning or stinging sensation, itching, mild redness of skin.

Severe: Rash, hives, skin blistering.

Storage and Administration

The oral medicine should be stored in a cool, dry place away from light. Prolonged exposure to heat, moisture, or light can damage the medicine.

The liquid may be stored at room temperature and does not need to be refrigerated.

The skin ointment, cream, and powder may be stored at room temperature.

Before the dose is measured, the liquid form of nystatin should be shaken well. The liquid should be swished around in the child's mouth for as long as she can before it is swallowed or spit out. This is called the "swish and swallow" or "swish and spit" method.

The powder should be mixed just before the dose is given. Do not store the mixed powder.

The lozenge must be dissolved slowly in the mouth—do not allow the child to swallow or chew it.

If the child is unable to swallow the nystatin tablet, it can be crushed and mixed with water or soft food (such as applesauce, pudding, jam, or jelly). This mixture should be swallowed and not chewed. The entire mixture must be swallowed to ensure that the child received the full dose.

Special Instructions

To obtain maximum benefit from the lozenge and liquid, do not allow the child to eat or drink for 30 minutes after each nystatin dose.

Skin ointment, cream, and powder are to be used only on the skin. Apply it carefully so it does not get into the child's eyes.

O xacillin sodium

Brand Names

Bactocill
(capsule)
Prostaphlin
(capsule,
liquid)

Common Uses

Oxacillin belongs to the class of medicines called antibiotics, which are used to treat a variety of bacterial infections. Oxacillin is prescribed for infections of the skin, soft tissue, respiratory tract, bone, and heart, because it prevents the bacteria from growing.

Oxacillin is effective only against bacterial infections, not those caused by viruses, parasites, or yeast.

Usual Dose

Children: 50–100 mg/kg/day divided into equal doses given every 6 hours.

Children who weigh more than 20 kg (44 lb) and Adults: 500–1000 mg/dose every 4–6 hours.

Medication Interactions

Medications that decrease the effectiveness of oxacillin are:

demeclocycline   minocycline

doxycycline   oxytetracycline

methacycline   tetracycline

Adverse Side Effects

Minor: Diarrhea, nausea, vomiting, heartburn, upset stomach, darkened tongue.

Severe: Rash, hives, difficulty breathing, blood in the urine, sore throat, fever, stomach cramps, seizures, yellow skin or eyes, unusual bleeding or bruising, severe diarrhea.

Storage and Administration

The oral medicine should be stored in a cool, dry place away from light. Prolonged exposure to heat, moisture, or light can damage the medicine.

Before the dose is measured, the liquid form of oxacillin should be shaken well. Refrigeration of the liquid is recommended. After receiving the liquid medicine from the pharmacy, it is good only for 14 days; therefore, always check the expiration date on the prescription label before using.

If the child is unable to swallow the capsule, it can be opened and mixed with water or a small amount of food (such as applesauce, pudding, jam, or jelly). This mixture should be swallowed and not chewed. The entire mixture must be swallowed to ensure that the child received the full dose.

Oxacillin works best when taken on an empty stomach (1 hour before a meal or 2–3 hours after a meal).

Special Instructions

The child's physician should be notified if the infection worsens or does not improve within 3–5 days.

N o t e s

O xybutynin

Brand Name

Ditropan
(tablet, liquid)

Common Uses

Oxybutynin belongs to the class of medicines called antispasmodics. Oxybutynin is used to decrease the number of times a person has to urinate, because it reduces the urge to urinate.

Usual Dose

Children 1–5 years old: 0.4–0.8 mg/kg/day divided into equal doses given 2–4 times a day.

Children older than 5 years: 10–15 mg/day divided into equal doses given 2–3 times a day.

Adults: 10–20 mg/day divided into equal doses given 2–4 times a day.

Medication Interactions

Oxybutynin may decrease the effectiveness of:

chlorpromazine	prochlorperazine
fluphenazine	promazine
haloperidol	promethazine
mesoridazine	thioridazine
perphenazine	trifluroperazine

Adverse Side Effects

Minor: Nausea, vomiting, constipation, bloating, blurred vision, dizziness, drowsiness, fatigue, headache, dry mouth, decreased sweating, insomnia, weakness, increased sensitivity of eyes to sunlight.

Severe: Rash, awareness of heartbeat, difficult or painful urination, eye pain, poor sight, hallucinations.

Storage and Administration

The oral medicine should be stored in a cool, dry place away from light. Prolonged exposure to heat, moisture, or light can damage the medicine.

The liquid may be stored at room temperature and does not need to be refrigerated.

If the child is unable to swallow the tablet, it can be crushed and mixed with water or soft food (such as applesauce, pudding, jam, or jelly). This mixture should be swallowed and not chewed. The entire mixture must be swallowed to ensure that the child received the entire dose.

If upset stomach occurs, oxybutynin can be given with food or milk.

Special Instructions

May cause drowsiness or dizziness in some people. Until it is known how the child will react to the medicine, activities that require mental alertness (such as physical education and playground activity) should be restricted.

For older children, dry mouth may be relieved by chewing gum or sucking on hard candy or ice chips. Younger children may need extra liquids.

The child may have to wear sunglasses outside, because oxybutynin may cause his eyes to become more sensitive to sunlight.

Oxybutynin increases the chance of heat stroke because it decreases the child's ability to sweat; therefore, physical education and playground activity should be restricted, especially on hot days.

N o t e s

P ancrelipase

Brand Names

Cotazym
(capsule)
Cotazym-S
(enteric-
coated
microspheres)
Ilozyme
(tablet)
Ku-Zyme
(tablet)
Pancrease
(enteric-
coated
microspheres)
Pancrease MT4
(enteric-
coated
microtablets)
Pancrease MT10
(enteric-
coated
microtablets)
Pancrease
MT16
(enteric-
coated
microtablets)
Protilase
(enteric-
coated
microspheres)
Ultrase MT20
(capsule)
Ultrase MT24
(capsule)
Viokase
(powder,
tablet)
Zymase
(enteric-
coated
microspheres)

Common Uses

Pancrelipase belongs to the class of medicines called digestive enzymes, which are used to replace naturally occurring digestive enzymes to help in the digestion and absorption of food in people with diseases that cause a lack of these enzymes.

Usual Dose

All doses given are suggested starting doses or dosage ranges. The dose is raised or lowered depending on the needs and response of each child.

POWDER

Children younger than 1 year old: One-eighth of a teaspoon (0.35 g) with all meals, feedings, and snacks. Maximum dose 6000 units of lipase/kg/dose.

ALL OTHER DOSAGE FORMS

Children 6 months–1 year old: 2,000 units of lipase given with all meals and feedings. Maximum dose 6000 units of lipase/kg/dose.

Children 1–6 years old: 4,000–8,000 units of lipase given with all meals and 4,000 units of lipase with all snacks. Maximum dose 6000 units of lipase/kg/dose.

Children 7–12 years old: 4,000–12,000 units of lipase given with all meals and snacks. Maximum dose 6000 units of lipase/kg/dose.

Children over 12 years and Adults: 4,000–48,000 units of lipase given with all meals and snacks. Maximum dose 6000 units of lipase/kg/dose.

Medication Interactions

Medications that may decrease the effectiveness of pancrelipase are:

antacids

iron salts

Adverse Side Effects

Minor: Nausea, upset stomach, diarrhea.

Severe: Blood in the urine, hives, joint pain, rash, swelling of the feet or legs, stomach pain.

Storage and Administration

The oral medicine should be stored in a cool, dry place away from light. Prolonged exposure to heat, moisture, or light can damage the medicine.

Give the child pancrelipase before meals, snacks, and feedings to obtain maximum benefit from the medicine.

Pancrelipase powder should be sprinkled over food.

Enteric-coated spheres should be swallowed whole. If the child is unable to do this, the spheres may be mixed with water or sprinkled over soft food (such as applesauce, pudding, jam, or jelly). This mixture should be swallowed and not chewed. The entire mixture must be swallowed to ensure that the child received the full dose.

Non–enteric-coated tablets can be crushed and sprinkled over soft food (such as applesauce, pudding, jam, or jelly).

Special Instructions

Be sure the child eats at the same time or shortly after taking this medicine. If no food is eaten, she may develop stomach pain and cramps.

N o t e s

P emoline

Brand Name

Cylert
(chewable
tablet, tablet)

Common Uses

Pemoline belongs to the class of medicines called stimulants, which are used to treat attention deficit disorder with hyperactivity (ADDH). Pemoline causes chemicals to be released into the brain that allow for more focused attention.

Usual Dose

Children 6 years and older: Start with 37.5 mg given as a single dose in the morning and increase dose as directed by the physician until the desired effect is achieved. Usual normal dosing range is 56.25–75 mg/day. Maximum dose 112.5 mg/day.

Medication Interactions

A medication that may increase the risk for the development of pemoline adverse side effects is:

loxapine

Pemoline may increase the risk for the development of adverse side effects of:

loxapine

Adverse Side Effects

Minor: Dizziness, drowsiness, headache, insomnia, irritability, loss of appetite, nausea, upset stomach.

Severe: Seizures; depression; hallucinations; rash; awareness of heartbeat; involuntary movement of the tongue, lips, hands, or feet; yellow skin or eyes.

Storage and Administration

The oral medicine should be stored in a cool, dry place away from light. Prolonged exposure to heat, moisture, or light can damage the medicine.

If upset stomach occurs, pemoline can be given with food.

The chewable tablet should be chewed thoroughly before it is swallowed.

If the child is unable to swallow the nonchewable tablet, it can be crushed and mixed with water or soft food (such as applesauce, pudding, jam, or jelly). This mixture should be swallowed and not chewed. The entire mixture must be swallowed to ensure that the child received the full dose.

Special Instructions

May cause dizziness or drowsiness in some people. Until it is known how the child will react to the medicine, activities that require mental alertness (such as physical education and playground activity) should be restricted.

Have the child avoid eating excessive amounts of chocolate or drinking beverages containing caffeine, because this may make him susceptible to insomnia, irritability, and hyperactivity.

Notes

Penicillin G potassium

Pentids (tablet, liquid)

Common Uses

Penicillin G potassium belongs to the class of medicines called antibiotics, which are used to treat a variety of bacterial infections. Penicillin G potassium is prescribed for infections of the middle ear, respiratory tract, and urinary tract, because it prevents the bacteria from growing.

Penicillin G potassium is effective only against bacterial infections, not those caused by viruses, parasites, or yeast.

Usual Dose

Children younger than 12 years: 25–50 mg/kg/day divided into equal doses given every 6–8 hours.

Children 12 years or older and Adults: 125–500 mg/dose given every 6–8 hours.

Doses of Penicillin G potassium may be given in "units" instead of "mg." Conversion for changing "mg" to "units" is 250 mg = 400,000 units.

Medication Interactions

Medications that decrease the effectiveness of penicillin G potassium are:

demeclocycline	minocycline
doxycycline	oxytetracycline
methacycline	tetracycline

Adverse Side Effects

Minor: Diarrhea, upset stomach, nausea, vomiting, heartburn, darkened tongue.

Severe: Rash, hives, difficulty breathing, blood in the urine, sore throat, fever, stomach cramps, seizures, unusual bleeding or bruising, severe diarrhea.

Storage and Administration

The oral medicine should be stored in a cool, dry place away from light. Prolonged exposure to heat, moisture, or light can damage the medicine.

Before the dose is measured, the liquid form of penicillin G potassium should be shaken well. Refrigeration of the liquid is recommended. After receiving the liquid medicine from the pharmacy, it is good only for 14 days; therefore, always check the expiration date on the prescription label before using.

If the child is unable to swallow the tablet, it can be crushed and mixed with water. The entire mixture must be swallowed to ensure that the child received the entire dose.

Do not allow the child to drink fruit juice or carbonated beverages 1 hour before or 1 hour after taking this medicine.

Penicillin G potassium should be taken on an empty stomach (1 hour before a meal or 2–3 hours after a meal).

Special Instructions

The child's physician should be notified if the infection worsens or does not improve within 3–5 days.

N o t e s

Penicillin V potassium

Brand Names

Beepen-VK
(tablet, liquid)

Betapen VK
(tablet, liquid)

Ledercillin VK
(tablet, liquid)

Penicillin VK
(tablet, liquid)

Pen-Vee K
(tablet, liquid)

Robicillin VK
(tablet)

V-cillin K
(tablet, liquid)

Veetids
(tablet, liquid)

Common Uses

Penicillin V potassium belongs to the class of medicines called antibiotics, which are used to treat a variety of bacterial infections. Penicillin V potassium can be used to treat infections of the middle ear, respiratory tract, urinary tract, skin, and sinuses, because it prevents the bacteria from growing. This medicine also can be used to prevent infections in certain children who are especially susceptible to infections.

Penicillin V potassium is effective only against bacterial infections, not those caused by viruses, parasites, or yeast.

Usual Dose

TREATMENT OF INFECTION

Children younger than 12 years: 25–50 mg/kg/day divided into equal doses given every 6–8 hours. Maximum dose 3 g/day.

Children 12 years or older and Adults: 125–500 mg/dose given every 6–8 hours.

PREVENTION OF INFECTION

Children younger than 5 years: 125 mg/dose given twice a day.

Children 5 years or older and Adults: 250 mg/dose given twice a day.

Doses of Penicillin V potassium may be given in "units" instead of "mg." Conversion for changing "mg" to "units" is 250 mg = 400,000 units.

Medication Interactions

Medications that decrease the effectiveness of penicillin V potassium are:

demeclocycline	minocycline
doxycycline	oxytetracycline
methacycline	tetracycline

Adverse Side Effects

Minor: Diarrhea, upset stomach, nausea, vomiting, heartburn, darkened tongue.

Severe: Rash, hives, difficulty breathing, blood in the urine, sore throat, fever, stomach cramps, seizures, unusual bleeding or bruising, severe diarrhea.

Storage and Administration

The oral medicine should be stored in a cool, dry place away from light. Prolonged exposure to heat, moisture, or light can damage the medicine.

Before the dose is measured, the liquid form of penicillin V potassium should be shaken well. Refrigeration of the liquid is recommended. After receiving the liquid medicine from the pharmacy, it is good only for 14 days; therefore, always check the expiration date on the prescription label before using.

Penicillin V potassium works best when taken on an empty stomach (1 hour before a meal or 2–3 hours after a meal), but if upset stomach occurs it can be given with food or milk.

If the child is unable to swallow the tablet, it can be crushed and mixed with a small amount of water or soft food (such as applesauce, pudding, jam, or jelly). This mixture should be swallowed and not chewed. The entire mixture must be swallowed to ensure that the child received the full dose.

Special Instructions

The child's physician should be notified if the infection worsens or does not improve within 3–5 days.

N o t e s

Permethrin

Brand Names

Elimit
  (skin cream)
Nix
  (hair liquid)

Common Uses

Permethrin belongs to both the scabicides and pediculicides classes of medicines. Permethrin is used to treat and prevent the spread of head lice and scabies, because it kills the live lice and scabies and their eggs.

Permethrin treats only head lice and scabies—not infections caused by bacteria, viruses, parasites, or yeast.

Usual Dose

SCABIES

CREAM: Apply to the entire body, from the head to the soles of the feet (for infants also apply to the hairline, scalp, neck, and forehead). Massage it into the skin, let it remain on the body for 8–14 hours, and then remove the cream with water.

HEAD LICE

HAIR LIQUID: Wash hair with shampoo, rinse, and towel dry. Apply permethrin to wet hair and leave in place for approximately 10 minutes, then rinse out with water. Use a special comb to remove the eggs.

Medication Interactions

No major medication interactions have been found with other oral medications.

Adverse Side Effects

Minor: Temporary skin itching, burning, stinging, numbness, or tingling.

Severe: Skin rash or swelling.

Storage and Administration

The skin cream and hair liquid should be stored in a cool, dry place away from light. Prolonged exposure to heat, moisture, or light can damage permethrin.

One application usually is enough to cure the infection. If another application is necessary, wait 7 days before reapplying permethrin.

Special Instructions

Skin cream and hair liquid are to be used only on the skin and hair; be careful not to get the medication into the child's eyes.

To remove all lice and scabies from bed linens, towels, and clothes, wash them in hot water or have them dry cleaned. Combs and brushes should be soaked in boiling water for 1 hour. This must be done the same day the medicine is applied to ensure that reinfection does not occur.

Notes

P henobarbital

Brand Name

Solfoton
(tablet,
capsule)

Generic
medicine
dosage form:
Phenobarbital
(tablet, liquid)

Common Uses

Phenobarbital belongs to the class of medicines called anticonvulsants. Phenobarbital decreases the ability of the seizure to spread throughout the brain.

Usual Dose

Children 1–5 years old: 6–8 mg/kg/day divided into equal doses given 1–2 times a day.

Children 6–12 years old: 4–6 mg/kg/day divided into equal doses given 1–2 times a day.

Children older than 12 years and Adults: 1–3 mg/kg/day divided into equal doses given 1–3 times a day.

Medication Interactions

A medication that may increase the risk for the development of phenobarbital adverse side effects is:

valproic acid

Phenobarbital may decrease the effectiveness of:

betamethasone	metoprolol
cortisone	metronidazole
dexamethasone	nifedipine
dicumarol	prednisolone
doxycycline	prednisone
felodipine	propranolol
fludrocortisone	quinidine
griseofulvin	theophylline
hydrocortisone	triamcinolone
methylprednisolone	warfarin

A medication that may cause severe drowsiness when combined with phenobarbital is:

alcohol

A medication that may cause increased risk of renal damage when combined with phenobarbital is:

methoxyflurane

Adverse Side Effects

Minor: Sedation, drowsiness, dizziness, diarrhea, nausea, upset stomach, headache, decreased attention span, hyperactivity in some children..

Severe: Sore throat, fever, unusual bruising or bleeding, difficulty breathing, chest pain, rash, hives, loss of coordination, slurred speech, yellow skin or eyes, hallucinations, joint or muscle pain, slow heartbeat, decreased learning ability.

Storage and Administration

The oral medicine should be stored in a cool, dry place away from light. Prolonged exposure to heat, moisture, or light can damage the medicine.

The liquid may be stored at room temperature and does not need to be refrigerated.

It is best to have the child take phenobarbital with food or milk to decrease or prevent stomach upset.

If the child is unable to swallow pills, the tablet can be crushed or the capsule opened and mixed with water or soft food (such as apple-sauce, pudding, jam, or jelly). This mixture should be swallowed and not chewed. The entire mixture must be swallowed to ensure that the child received the full dose.

Special Instructions

May cause sedation, drowsiness, and dizziness in some people. Until it is known how the child will react to the medicine, activities that require mental alertness (such as physical education and playground activity) should be restricted.

Some studies have shown that children taking phenobarbital for seizures have more difficulty learning. These children may need extra help with their learning activities if they are having such difficulties.

Do not suddenly stop giving phenobarbital to the child unless instructed to do so by a physician. Suddenly stopping this medication may cause severe seizures to occur.

P henylpropanolamine hydrochloride

Brand Names

Propagest
(tablet)
Rhindecon
(long-acting
capsule)

Common Uses

Phenylpropanolamine belongs to the class of medicines called decongestants. Decongestants are used to treat nasal congestion caused by the common cold, hay fever, and respiratory allergies. They reduce congestion by narrowing the blood vessels in the nose.

Usual Dose

Children 2–6 years old: 6.25 mg/dose given every 4 hours.

Children 6–12 years old: 12.5 mg/dose given every 4 hours. Maximum dose 75 mg/day.

Children older than 12 years and Adults

TABLET: 25 mg/dose given every 4 hours. Maximum dose 150 mg/day.

LONG-ACTING CAPSULE: 75 mg/dose given every 12 hours. Maximum dose 150 mg/day.

Medication Interactions

A medication that may increase the risk for the development of phenylpropanolamine adverse side effects is:

furazolidone

A medication that may decrease the effectiveness of phenylpropanolamine is:

guanethidine

Phenylpropanolamine may decrease the effectiveness of:

guanethidine

Medications that may cause severe headaches, dangerous increases in body temperature, or increased blood pressure when combined with phenylpropanolamine are:

isocarboxazid	phenelzine
pargyline	tranylcypromine

Adverse Side Effects

Minor: Nausea, vomiting, dizziness, headache, nervousness, loss of appetite, insomnia.

Severe: Tightness in the chest, awareness of heartbeat, fast heartbeat, irregular or unusual heartbeat, high blood pressure.

Storage and Administration

The oral medicine should be stored in a cool, dry place away from light. Prolonged exposure to heat, moisture, or light can damage the medicine.

If upset stomach occurs, phenylpropanolamine can be given with food or milk.

The long-acting capsule should be swallowed whole with a full glass of water. Do not crush or allow the child to chew it.

If the child is unable to swallow the tablet, it can be crushed and mixed with soft food (such as applesauce, pudding, jam, or jelly). This mixture should be swallowed and not chewed. The entire mixture must be swallowed to ensure that the child received the full dose.

Special Instructions

Do not allow the child to drink products containing caffeine, because caffeine-related side effects (headache, trembling, nervousness, insomnia, fast heartbeat) are more likely to occur.

May cause dizziness in some people. Until it is known how the child will react to the medicine, activities that require mental alertness (such as physical education and playground activity) should be restricted.

N o t e s

Phenytoin sodium

Dilantin 30
  Pediatric
  (liquid)

Dilantin 125
  (liquid)

Dilantin Infatab
  (chewable
  tablet)

Dilantin
  Kapseals
  (long-acting
  capsule)

Diphenylan
  sodium
  (capsule)

Common Uses

Phenytoin belongs to the class of medicines called anticonvulsants. Phenytoin decreases the ability of the seizure to spread throughout the brain.

Usual Dose

Children 6 months–3 years old: 8–10 mg/kg/day divided into equal doses given every 8–12 hours.

Children 4–6 years old: 7.5–9 mg/kg/day divided into equal doses given every 8–12 hours.

Children 7–9 years old: 7–8 mg/kg/day divided into equal doses given every 8–12 hours.

Children 10–16 years old: 6–7 mg/kg/day divided into equal doses given every 8–12 hours.

Adults: 4–7 mg/kg/day or 300–400 mg/day divided into equal doses given 2–3 times a day, or 1–2 times a day if the long-acting capsule is given.

Medication Interactions

Medications that may increase the risk for the development of phenytoin adverse side effects are:

amiodarone	sulfadiazine
chloramphenicol	sulfamethizole
cimetidine	trimethoprim
dicumarol	trimethoprim
disulfiram	with sulfamethoxazole
fluconazole	valproic acid
isoniazid	warfarin

Medications that may decrease the effectiveness of phenytoin are:

carbamazepine	rifabutin

P

dexamethasone	rifampin
diazoxide	sucralfate
folic acid	theophylline

Phenytoin may increase the risk for the development of adverse side effects of:

acetaminophen	primidone
chloramphenicol	warfarin
dicumarol	zalcitabine
disopyramide	

Phenytoin may decrease the effectiveness of:

acetaminophen	hydrocortisone
betamethasone	methadone
carbamazepine	methylprednisolone
chloramphenicol	metyrapone
cortisone	mexiletine
cyclosporine	prednisolone
dexamethasone	prednisone
disopyramide	quinidine
doxycycline	theophylline
felodipine	triamcinolone
fludrocortisone	valproic acid
furosemide	

Adverse Side Effects

Minor: Drowsiness, dizziness, headache, insomnia, nausea, constipation, increased amount of body or facial hair.

Severe: Sore throat, fever, unusual bruising or bleeding, yellow skin or eyes, hallucinations, slurred speech, rash, blurred or double vision, joint pain, bleeding gums, swollen or tender gums.

P

Storage and Administration

The oral medicine should be stored in a cool, dry place away from light. Prolonged exposure to heat, moisture, or light can damage the medicine.

Before the dose is measured, the liquid form of phenytoin should be shaken well. The liquid may be stored at room temperature and does not need to be refrigerated.

It is best to give phenytoin with food or milk to decrease or prevent upset stomach.

The chewable tablet should be chewed thoroughly before swallowing.

The long-acting capsule should be swallowed whole with a full glass of water. Do not crush or allow the child to chew it.

If the child is unable to swallow the non–long-acting capsule, it can be opened and mixed with a small amount of soft food (such as applesauce, pudding, jam, or jelly). This mixture should be swallowed and not chewed. The entire mixture must be swallowed to ensure that the child received the full dose.

Special Instructions

May cause sedation, drowsiness, and dizziness in some people. Until it is known how the child will react to the medicine, activities that require mental alertness (such as physical education and playground activity) should be restricted.

Do not suddenly stop giving phenytoin to the child unless instructed to do so by a physician. Suddenly stopping this medication may cause severe seizures to occur.

The child should brush and floss her teeth and massage the gums regularly and carefully. The dentist should be visited regularly.

N o t e s

Prednisolone P

Common Uses

Prednisolone belongs to the class of medicines called corticosteroids, which are used to treat asthma, allergies, inflammatory diseases, and various other problems. Prednisolone affects many different substances in the body that may cause or worsen these conditions

Usual Dose

Children: 0.1–2 mg/kg/day divided into equal doses given 1–4 times a day.

Adults: 5–60 mg/day divided into equal doses given 1–4 times a day.

Medication Interactions

Medications that may increase the risk for the development of prednisolone adverse side effects are:

conjugated estrogen	ketoconazole
estradiol	mestranol
estriol	troleandomycin
ethinyl estradiol	

Medications that may decrease the effectiveness of prednisolone are:

phenobarbital	primidone
phenytoin	rifampin

Prednisolone may decrease the effectiveness of:

aspirin	magnesium salicylate
bismuth subsalicylate	salsalate
choline salicylate	sodium salicylate

Adverse Side Effects

Minor: Round face, weight gain, acne, upset stomach, nausea, vomiting, increased appetite, dizziness.

Brand Names

Delta-Cortef
(tablet)
Pediapred
(liquid)
Prelone (liquid)

P

Severe: Rash; difficulty swallowing; hives; increased thirst; headache; seizures; insomnia; fatigue; dizziness; black, tarry stools; sore throat; fever; hallucinations; irregular heartbeat; blurred vision; stomach pain; nightmares; difficulty breathing; leg cramps.

Storage and Administration

The oral medicine should be stored in a cool, dry place away from light. Prolonged exposure to heat, moisture, or light can damage the medicine.

The liquid may be stored at room temperature and does not need to be refrigerated.

It is best to give prednisolone with food or milk to decrease or prevent upset stomach.

If the child is unable to swallow the tablet, it can be crushed and mixed with soft food (such as applesauce, pudding, jam, or jelly). This mixture should be swallowed and not chewed. The entire mixture must be swallowed to ensure that the child received the full dose.

Special Instructions

May cause dizziness in some people. Until it is known how the child will react to the medicine, activities that require mental alertness (such as physical education and playground activity) should be restricted.

If the child has been taking prednisolone for more than 1 week, do not abruptly stop it. Suddenly stopping the oral medicine (tablet and liquid) can cause nausea, vomiting, weakness, fever, shortness of breath, stomach or back pain, or dizziness.

If the child has been taking prednisolone for more than 1 week, notify the physician who prescribed the prednisolone if a serious injury or illness occurs.

The child's physician should be notified at once if there is blood in the urine or black, tarry stools.

Prednisone P

Common Uses

Prednisone belongs to the class of medicines called corticosteroids, which are used to treat asthma, allergies, inflammatory diseases, and various other problems. Prednisone affects many different substances in the body that may cause or worsen these conditions.

Usual Dose

Children: 0.05–2 mg/kg/day divided into equal doses given 1–4 times a day.

Adults: 5–60 mg/day divided into equal doses given 1–4 times a day.

Medication Interactions

Medications that may increase the risk for the development of prednisone adverse side effects are:

conjugated estrogen	ketoconazole
estradiol	mestranol
estriol	troleandomycin
ethinyl estradiol	

Medications that may decrease the effectiveness of prednisone are:

phenobarbital	primidone
phenytoin	rifampin

Prednisone may decrease the effectiveness of:

aspirin	magnesium salicylate
bismuth subsalicylate	salsalate
choline salicylate	sodium salicylate

Adverse Side Effects

Minor: Round face, weight gain, acne, upset stomach, nausea, vomiting, increased appetite, dizziness.

Brand Names

Deltasone
(tablet)

Liquid Pred
(liquid)

Meticorten
(tablet)

Orasone
(tablet)

Panasol-S
(tablet)

Prednicen-M
(tablet)

Prednisone
Intensol
(concentrate)

Sterapred
(tablet)

Sterapred DS
(tablet)

P

Severe: Rash; difficulty swallowing; hives; increased thirst; headache; seizures; insomnia; fatigue; dizziness; black, tarry stools; blood in the urine; sore throat; fever; hallucinations; irregular heartbeat; blurred vision; stomach pain; nightmares; difficulty breathing; leg cramps.

Storage and Administration

The oral medicine should be stored in a cool, dry place away from light. Prolonged exposure to heat, moisture, or light can damage the medicine.

The liquid and concentrate may be stored at room temperature and do not need to be refrigerated.

The prednisone concentrate should be mixed with half a cup or more of fruit juice, milk, water, or carbonated beverage, or with a small amount of soft food (such as applesauce, pudding, jam, or jelly). Prepare the mixture just before giving the dose. The medicine will be damaged if left in the mixture; therefore, do not premix and store.

It is best to give prednisone with food or milk to decrease or prevent upset stomach.

If the child is unable to swallow the tablet, it can be crushed and mixed with soft food (such as applesauce, pudding, jam, or jelly). This mixture should be swallowed and not chewed. The entire mixture must be swallowed to ensure that the child received the full dose.

Special Instructions

May cause dizziness in some people. Until it is known how the child will react to the medicine, activities that require mental alertness (such as physical education and playground activity) should be restricted.

If the child has been taking prednisone for more than 1 week, do not abruptly stop giving the drug. Suddenly stopping the oral medicine (tablet, liquid, or concentrate) can cause nausea, vomiting, weakness, fever, shortness of breath, stomach or back pain, or dizziness.

If the child has been taking prednisone for more than 1 week, notify the physician who prescribed the prednisone if a serious injury or illness occurs.

The child's physician should be notified at once if there is blood in the urine or black, tarry stools.

Primidone

Common Uses

Primidone belongs to the class of medicines called anticonvulsants. Primidone decreases the ability of the seizure to spread throughout the brain.

Usual Dose

Children younger than 8 years: Start with 50–125 mg/dose given once a day. Increase the dose according to the physician's directions to a dose of 10–25 mg/kg/ day divided into equal doses given 3–4 times a day.

Children 8 years or older and Adults: Start with 125–250 mg/dose given once a day. Increase the dose according to the physician's directions to a dose of 750–1500 mg/day divided into equal doses given 3–4 times a day. Maximum dose 2 g/day.

Medication Interactions

Medications that may increase the risk for the development of primidone adverse side effects are:

phenytoin

valproic acid

Medications that may decrease the effectiveness of primidone are:

ethosuximide

methsuximide

Primidone may decrease the effectiveness of:

betamethasone	metoprolol
cortisone	nifedipine
dexamethasone	prednisolone
dicumarol	prednisone
doxycycline	propranolol

Brand Name

Mysoline
(tablet, liquid)

P

felodipine   quinidine

fludrocortisone   theophylline

griseofulvin   triamcinolone

hydrocortisone   warfarin

methylprednisolone

A medication that may cause increased risk of kidney damage when combined with primidone is:

methoxyflurane

Adverse Side Effects

Minor: Dizziness, drowsiness, headache, fatigue, nausea.

Severe: Difficulty breathing, blurred or double vision, unusual eye movements, rash, hives, irritability, agitation, fever, sore throat, joint pain.

Storage and Administration

The oral medicine should be stored in a cool, dry place away from light. Prolonged exposure to heat, moisture, or light can damage the medicine.

Before the dose is measured, the liquid form of primidone should be shaken well. The liquid may be stored at room temperature and does not need to be refrigerated.

If upset stomach occurs, the medicine can be given with food or milk.

If the child is unable to swallow the primidone tablet, it can be crushed and mixed with water or juice. The entire mixture must be swallowed to ensure that the child received the full dose.

Special Instructions

May cause sedation, drowsiness, and dizziness in some people. Until it is known how the child will react to the medicine, activities that require mental alertness (such as physical education and playground activity) should be restricted.

Do not suddenly stop giving primidone to the child unless instructed to do so by a physician. Suddenly stopping this medication may cause severe seizures to occur.

Procainamide hydrochloride

Common Uses

Procainamide belongs to the class of medicines called antiarrhythmics. Procainamide slows electrical impulses that cause the heart to beat in an irregular rhythm.

Usual Dose

Children: 15–50 mg/kg/day divided into equal doses given every 3–6 hours. Maximum dose 4 g/day.

Adults

TABLET AND CAPSULE: 250–500 mg/dose given every 3–6 hours. Maximum dose 4 g/day.

LONG-ACTING TABLET: 2–4 g/day divided into equal doses given every 6 hours. Maximum dose 4 g/day.

Medication Interactions

Medications that may increase the risk for the development of procainamide adverse side effects are:

amiodarone

cimetidine

trimethoprim

Adverse Side Effects

Minor: Diarrhea, upset stomach, nausea, vomiting, bad taste in mouth, dry mouth, dizziness, headache, loss of appetite.

Severe: Stomach pain, chest pain, chills, fatigue, fever, sore throat or mouth, hallucinations, confusion, depression, rash, muscle or joint pain, itching, awareness of heartbeat, abnormal heartbeat, seizures, unusual bruising or bleeding, yellow skin or eyes.

Storage and Administration

The oral medicine should be stored in a cool, dry place away from light. Prolonged exposure to heat, moisture, or light can damage the medicine.

Brand Names

Procan SR
 (long-acting
 tablet)

Pronestyl
 (tablet,
 capsule)

Pronestyl-SR
 (long-acting
 tablet)

P

Procainamide works best when taken on an empty stomach (1 hour before a meal or 2–3 hours after a meal), but if upset stomach occurs it can be given with food.

The long-acting tablet should be swallowed whole with a full glass of water. Do not crush or allow the child to chew it.

If the child is unable to swallow pills, the non–long-acting tablet can be crushed or the capsule opened and mixed with a small amount of water or soft food (such as applesauce, pudding, jam, or jelly). This mixture should be swallowed and not chewed. The entire mixture must be swallowed to ensure that the child received the full dose.

Special Instructions

May cause dizziness in some people. Until it is known how the child will react to the medicine, activities that require mental alertness (such as physical education and playground activity) should be restricted.

For older children, dry mouth may be relieved by chewing gum or sucking on hard candy or ice chips. Younger children may need extra liquids.

The empty long-acting tablet may be seen in the stool. This is normal and no extra doses are needed.

Notes

Promethazine hydrochloride

Common Uses

Promethazine belongs to the class of medicines called antihistamines. Promethazine is used to treat seasonal and constant runny nose and sneezing caused by allergies and colds, because It blocks the chemical histamine, which causes these problems. Promethazine also is used to prevent motion sickness, and to control or prevent vomiting.

Usual Dose

ALLERGIES AND COLDS

TABLET, LIQUID, AND RECTAL SUPPOSITORY

Children: 0.1 mg/kg/dose given every 6 hours during the day and 0.5 mg/kg/dose at bedtime.

Adults: 12.5 mg/dose given every 8 hours during the day and 25 mg/dose at bedtime.

MOTION SICKNESS

TABLET, LIQUID, AND RECTAL SUPPOSITORY

Children: 0.5 mg/kg/dose given every 12 hours.

or

12.5–25 mg/dose given every 12 hours.

Adults: 25 mg/dose given every 12 hours.

VOMITING

TABLET, LIQUID, AND RECTAL SUPPOSITORY

Children: 0.25–1 mg/kg/dose given every 4–6 hours as needed to control vomiting.

Adults: 12.5–25 mg/kg/dose given every 4 hours as needed to control vomiting.

Medication Interactions

Medications that may increase the risk for the development of promethazine adverse side effects are:

alcohol	oxybutynin
atropine	scopolamine
benztropine	trihexyphenidyl

Brand Names

Phenameth
(tablet)

Phenergan
(tablet, liquid,
rectal
suppository)

P

A medication that may cause severe drowsiness when combined with promethazine is:

alcohol

Adverse Side Effects

Minor: Drowsiness, dizziness, dry mouth, headache, nausea, diarrhea, increased sensitivity to sunlight.

Severe: Confusion; excitability; weakness; blurred vision; involuntary movement of the face, mouth, and tongue; rash; yellow skin or eyes; unusual bruising or bleeding.

Storage and Administration

The oral medicine should be stored in a cool, dry place away from light. Prolonged exposure to heat, moisture, or light can damage the medicine.

The liquid may be stored at room temperature and does not need to be refrigerated.

Refrigeration of the rectal suppository is recommended.

If upset stomach occurs, promethazine can be given with food.

Do not crush the tablet because of the bad taste of the powder.

Special Instructions

May cause sedation, drowsiness, and dizziness in some people. Until it is known how the child will react to the medicine, activities that require mental alertness (such as physical education and playground activity) should be restricted.

May cause dizziness or upon standing; therefore, always have the child stand up slowly. If the child becomes dizzy, she should be instructed to sit or lie down immediately.

Have the child avoid prolonged exposure to sunlight, because this medication may cause her to be more sensitive to it.

For older children, dry mouth may be relieved by chewing gum or sucking on hard candy or ice chips. Younger children may need extra liquids.

Propranolol hydrochloride

Common Uses

Propranolol belongs to the class of medicines called beta-blockers. Propranolol is used to treat and control high blood pressure, prevent chest pain, and keep the heart beating at a regular rate and rhythm. It blocks specific impulses that may cause or worsen these conditions. Propranolol also can be used to prevent migraine headaches.

Usual Dose

ABNORMAL HEARTBEAT

Children: 0.5–4 mg/kg/day divided into equal doses given every 6–8 hours. Maximum dose 16 mg/kg/day or 60 mg/day.

Adults: 10–30 mg/dose given 3–4 times a day.

HIGH BLOOD PRESSURE

Children: 0.5–2 mg/kg/day divided into equal doses given every 6–12 hours.

Adults

TABLET AND LIQUID: 80–240 mg/day divided into equal doses given 2–3 times a day. Maximum dose 640 mg/day.

LONG-ACTING CAPSULE: 80–160 mg/dose given once a day. Maximum dose 640 mg/day.

MIGRAINE HEADACHE

Children who weigh 35 kg or less (77 lb): 10–20 mg/dose given 3 times a day.

Children who weigh more than 35 kg: 20–40 mg/dose given 3 times a day.

Adults

TABLET AND LIQUID: 80–240 mg/day divided into equal doses given every 6–8 hours. Maximum dose 320 mg/day.

LONG-ACTING TABLET: 80–240 mg/day given once a day. Maximum dose 320 mg/day.

Brand Names

Inderal
  (tablet)

Inderal LA
  (long-acting
  capsule)

Propranolol
Intensol
  (concentrate)

Generic
  medicine
  dosage form:
  Propranolol
  (tablet, long-
  acting
  capsule,
  liquid)

P

Medication Interactions

Medications that may increase the risk for the development of propranolol adverse side effects are:

cimetidine	propylthiouracil
hydralazine	propafenone
methimazole	verapamil

Medications that decrease the effectiveness of propranolol are:

phenobarbital	indomethacin
primidone	piroxicam
ibuprofen	rifampin

Propranolol increases the risk for the development of adverse side effects of:

chlorpromazine	thioridazine
hydralazine	verapamil

Propranolol decreases the effectiveness of:

clonidine

theophylline

Medications that may cause the arms and legs to become cold when combined with propranolol are:

dihydroergotamine	methysergide
ergotamine	theophylline

A medication that may increase the risk of dizziness upon standing when combined with propranolol is:

prazosin

Propranolol may hide the symptoms of low blood sugar when combined with:

insulin

Adverse Side Effects

Minor: Constipation; diarrhea; nausea; upset stomach; dizziness; drowsiness; dry mouth, eyes, or skin; headache; fatigue, weakness.

Severe: Difficulty breathing, wheezing, chest pain, cold hands or feet, hallucinations, nightmares, insomnia, numbness or tingling in the fingers or toes, fever, sore throat, sudden weight gain (3–5 lb), swelling of the legs or feet, joint pain, unusual bruising or bleeding, prolonged fatigue, slow heartbeat.

Storage and Administration

The oral medicine should be stored in a cool, dry place away from light. Prolonged exposure to heat, moisture, or light can damage the medicine.

The liquid and concentrate may be stored at room temperature and do not need to be refrigerated.

The concentrate should be mixed with half a cup or more of fruit juice, milk, water, or carbonated beverage, or with soft food (such as applesauce, pudding, jam, or jelly). Prepare the mixture just before giving the dose. The medicine will be damaged if left in the mixture; therefore, do not premix and store.

It is best to give propranolol with food or milk to increase the amount of medicine that the body absorbs.

The long-acting capsule should be swallowed whole with a full glass of water. Do not crush or allow the child to chew it.

If the child is unable to swallow the tablet, it can be crushed and mixed with water, juice, or soft food (such as applesauce, pudding, jam, or jelly). This mixture should be swallowed and not chewed. The entire mixture must be swallowed to ensure that the child received the full dose.

Special Instructions

May cause drowsiness or dizziness in some people. Until it is known how the child will react to the medicine, activities that require mental alertness (such as physical education and playground activity) should be restricted.

May cause dizziness upon standing; therefore, always have the child stand up slowly. If the child becomes dizzy, he should be instructed to sit or lie down immediately.

For older children, dry mouth may be relieved by chewing gum or sucking on hard candy or ice chips. Younger children may need extra liquids.

P

Dry eyes may be relieved by using artificial tears.

Propranolol may cause asthma attacks in children with asthma, even if the child's condition is currently controlled.

In children with diabetes, propranolol may mask the signs of hypo-glycemia (low blood sugar).

It is very important that this medicine is not suddenly stopped; to do so would cause the child's blood pressure to become very high.

N o t e s

Pseudoephedrine hydrochloride

Common Uses

Pseudoephedrine belongs to the class of medicines called decongestants, which are used to treat nasal congestion caused by common cold, hay fever, and respiratory allergies. Pseudoephedrine reduces congestion by narrowing the blood vessels in the nose.

Usual Dose

TABLET AND LIQUID

Children younger than 2 years: 4 mg/kg/day divided into equal doses given every 4–6 hours.

Children 2–5 years old: 15 mg/dose given every 4–6 hours. Maximum dose 60 mg/day.

Children 6–12 years old: 30 mg/dose given every 4–6 hours. Maximum dose 120 mg/day.

Children older than 12 years and Adults: 30–60 mg/dose given every 4–6 hours. Maximum dose 240 mg/day.

LONG-ACTING TABLET

Children older than 12 years and Adults: 120 mg/dose given every 12 hours.

Medication Interactions

Medications that may increase the risk for the development of pseudoephedrine adverse side effects are:

furazolidone   sodium bicarbonate

methyldopa   sodium citrate

potassium citrate   sodium lactate

sodium acetate

Brand Names

Allermed
(capsule)

Cenafed
(tablet, liquid)

Children's
Sudafed
(liquid)

Decofed
(liquid)

Dorcol
Children's
Decongestant
(liquid)

Genaphed
(tablet)

Halofed
(tablet)

Novafed
(long-acting
tablet)

PediaCare
Infant's
Decongestant
(liquid)

Pseudo
(liquid)

Pseudo-Gest
(tablet)

Sinustop Pro
(capsule)

Sudafed
(tablet)

Sudafed 12
hours
(long-acting
tablet)

P

A medication that may decrease the effectiveness of pseudo-ephedrine is:

guanethidine

Pseudoephedrine may decrease the effectiveness of:

guanethidine

Medications that may cause severe headaches, dangerous increases in body temperature, or increased blood pressure when combined with pseudoephedrine are:

isocarboxazid	phenelzine
pargyline	tranylcypromine

Adverse Side Effects

Minor: Agitation, insomnia, dizziness, headache, weakness.

Severe: Hallucinations, seizures, irregular or slow heartbeat, awareness of heartbeat, difficulty breathing, trembling, sweating.

Storage and Administration

The oral medicine should be stored in a cool, dry place away from light. Prolonged exposure to heat, moisture, or light can damage the medicine.

The liquid may be stored at room temperature and does not need to be refrigerated.

The long-acting tablet should be swallowed whole with a full glass of water. Do not crush or chew.

If the child is unable to swallow pills, the non–long-acting tablet may be crushed or the capsule may be opened and mixed with water, fruit juice, or soft food (such as applesauce, pudding, jam, or jelly). This mixture should be swallowed and not chewed. The entire mixture must be swallowed to ensure that the child received the entire dose.

If upset stomach occurs, pseudoephedrine can be given with food.

Special Instructions

May cause dizziness in some people. Until it is known how the child will react to the medicine, activities that require mental alertness (such as physical education and playground activity) should be restricted.

N o t e s

P yrazinamide

None

Generic medicine dosage form: Pyrazinamide (tablet)

Common Uses

Pyrazinamide belongs to the class of medicines called antituberculars. Pyrazinamide is used to treat tuberculosis, because it prevents the bacteria from growing.

Pyrazinamide is effective only against tuberculosis, not infections caused by other bacteria, viruses, parasites, or yeast.

Usual Doses

Children: 15–30 mg/kg/day divided into equal doses given 1–2 times a day or 50 mg/kg/dose given twice a week. Maximum dose 2 g/day.

Adults: 15–30 mg/kg/day divided into equal doses given once a day or 3–4 times a day. Maximum dose 3 g/day or 2 g/day if given once a day.

or

50–70 mg/kg/dose given twice a week. Maximum dose 3 g/day.

Medication Interactions

No major medication interactions have been found with other oral medications.

Adverse Side Effects

Minor: Nausea, vomiting, increased sensitivity to sunlight.

Severe: Stomach pain, fever, sore throat, fatigue, joint pain or inflammation, rash, loss of appetite, dark urine, joint or muscle pain, unusual bruising or bleeding, yellow skin or eyes.

Storage and Administration

The oral medicine should be stored in a cool, dry place away from light. Prolonged exposure to heat, moisture, or light can damage the medicine.

If upset stomach occurs, pyrazinamide can be given with food or milk.

If the child is unable to swallow the tablet, it can be crushed and mixed with a small amount of water or soft food (such as applesauce, pudding, jam, or jelly). This mixture should be swallowed and not chewed. The entire mixture must be swallowed to ensure that the child received the full dose.

Special Instructions

The child's physician should be notified if the infection worsens or does not improve within 2–3 weeks.

Have the child avoid prolonged exposure to sunlight, because this medication may cause him to be more sensitive to it.

N o t e s

R anitidine

Zantac
(tablet, liquid)

Common Uses

Ranitidine belongs to the class of medicines called histamine$_2$-antagonists. Ranitidine is used to treat and prevent certain types of stomach and upper intestine ulcers. Ranitidine also is used in diseases in which there is too much acid in the stomach (hypersecretory conditions) and when the airway is hurt by stomach acid (gastroesophageal reflux). Ranitidine reduces the amount of acid in the stomach by blocking the chemical histamine, which is responsible for secretion of acid into the stomach.

Usual Dose

Children: 1.25–2.5 mg/kg/dose given every 12 hours. Maximum dose 300 mg/day.

Adults

ULCER PREVENTION: 150 mg/dose given at bedtime.

ULCER TREATMENT: 150 mg/dose given every 12 hours or 300 mg/dose at bedtime.

HYPERSECRETORY CONDITIONS: 150 mg/dose given twice a day. Doses up to 6 g/day have been used.

GASTROESOPHAGEAL REFLUX: 150 mg/dose given twice a day.

Medication Interactions

Ranitidine may decrease the effectiveness of:

ketoconazole

A medication that may cause drowsiness, sedation, or lack of coordination when combined with ranitidine is:

alcohol

Adverse Side Effects

Minor: Nausea, diarrhea, constipation, upset stomach, dizziness, headache.

Severe: Rash; confusion; hallucinations; fatigue; unusual bruising or bleeding; black, tarry stools; vomiting that looks like coffee grounds.

Storage and Administration

The oral medicine should be stored in a cool, dry place away from light. Prolonged exposure to heat, moisture, or light can damage the medicine.

The liquid may be stored at room temperature and does not need to be refrigerated.

If the child is unable to swallow the tablet, it can be crushed and mixed with a small amount of water or soft food (such as applesauce, pudding, jam, or jelly). This mixture should be swallowed and not chewed. The entire mixture must be swallowed to ensure that the child received the full dose.

If upset stomach occurs, ranitidine can be given with food or milk.

Do not allow the child to take antacids within 1 hour before or 1 hour after taking ranitidine.

Special Instructions

May cause dizziness in some people. Until it is known how the child will react to the medicine, activities that require mental alertness (such as physical education and playground activity) should be restricted.

The child's physician should be notified as soon as possible if vomiting that looks like coffee grounds or black, tarry stools occur.

N o t e s

R ifampin

Brand Names

Rifadin
(capsule)
Rimactane
(capsule)

Common Uses

Rifampin belongs to the class of medicines called antituberculars. Rifampin is primarily used to treat tuberculosis. Rifampin also can be prescribed to treat infections of the skin and bones, and to prevent the spread of certain diseases. Rifampin is effective against these infections because it prevents the bacteria from growing.

Rifampin is effective only against bacterial infections, not those caused by viruses, parasites, or yeast.

Usual Dose

TUBERCULOSIS

Children: 10–20 mg/kg/day divided into equal doses given 1–2 times a day. Maximum dose 600 mg/day.

or

10–20 mg/kg/dose given twice a week. Maximum dose 600 mg/dose.

Adults: 10 mg/kg/dose given once a day or twice a week. Maximum dose 600 mg/dose.

PREVENTION

Infants and Children: 20 mg/kg/day divided into equal doses given every 12–24 hours. Maximum dose 600 mg/dose.

Adults: 600 mg/dose given every 12–24 hours.

Medication Interactions

A medication that may decrease the effectiveness of rifampin is:

ketoconazole

Rifampin may decrease the effectiveness of:

acetohexamide

betamethasone

chlorpropamide

cyclosporine

dexamethasone

dicumarol

disopyramide

fludrocortisone

glipizide

glyburide

hydrocortisone

ketoconazole

methylprednisolone

metoprolol

phenytoin

prednisolone

prednisone

propranolol

quinidine

theophylline

tolazamide

tolbutamide

triamcinolone

verapamil

warfarin

A medication that may increase the risk for the development of liver toxicity when combined with rifampin is:

isoniazid

Adverse Side Effects

Minor: Nausea; vomiting; diarrhea; upset stomach; dizziness; drowsiness; headache; heartburn; loss of appetite; reddish-brown to reddish-orange urine, stools, tears, sweat, and saliva.

Severe: Fatigue; confusion; stomach cramps; fever; chills; sore throat, mouth, or tongue; blurred vision or other visual problems; rash; muscle pain or weakness; uncontrolled movements; painful arms or legs; difficult or painful urination; difficulty breathing; unusual bruising or bleeding; yellow skin or eyes.

Storage and Administration

The oral medicine should be stored in a cool, dry place away from light. Prolonged exposure to heat, moisture, or light can damage the medicine.

R

Rifampin works best when taken on an empty stomach (1 hour before a meal or 2–3 hours after a meal), but if upset stomach occurs it can be given with food.

If the child is unable to swallow the capsule, it can be opened and mixed with water or a small amount of soft food (such as applesauce, pudding, jam, or jelly). This mixture should be swallowed and not chewed. The entire mixture must be swallowed to ensure that the child received the full dose.

Special Instructions

May cause drowsiness or dizziness in some people. Until it is known how the child will react to the medicine, activities that require mental alertness (such as physical education and playground activity) should be restricted.

May cause the urine, stool, tears, sweat, and saliva to become reddish-brown to reddish-orange in color. This effect occurs often and is harmless.

Do not allow the child to wear soft contact lenses while taking rifampin, because they will become permanently stained if the tears turn color. No time frame has been specified as to when the child could start wearing the lenses again; however, waiting 7 days probably would be safe.

N o t e s

Rimantadine hydrochloride

Common Uses

Rimantadine belongs to the class of medicines called antivirals. Rimantadine is prescribed for viral infections of the respiratory tract caused by influenza. Rimantadine is effective against these infections because it prevents the virus from growing.

Rimantadine is effective only against infections caused by the influenza virus, not those caused by other viruses, bacteria, parasites, or yeast.

Usual Dose

Children younger than 10 years: 5 mg/kg/dose given once a day. Maximum dose 150 mg/dose.

Children 10 years or older and Adults: 100 mg/dose given 2 times a day.

Medication Interactions

A medication that may increase the risk for the development of rimantadine adverse side effects is:

cimetidine

Medications that may decrease the effectiveness of rimantadine are:

acetaminophen

aspirin

Adverse Side Effects

Minor: Nausea, vomiting, upset stomach, diarrhea, constipation, dizziness, headache, nervousness, fatigue, dry mouth, decreased concentration.

Severe: Hallucinations, difficulty breathing, seizures, awareness of heartbeat, fast heartbeat, pale skin, fever, chills, confusion, difficult or painful swallowing.

Brand Name

Flumadine
(tablet, liquid)

Storage and Administration

The oral medicine should be stored in a cool, dry place away from light. Prolonged exposure to heat, moisture, or light can damage the medicine.

The liquid may be stored at room temperature and does not need to be refrigerated.

If upset stomach occurs, rimantadine can be given with food.

If the child is unable to swallow the tablet, it can be crushed and mixed with water or soft food (such as applesauce, pudding, jam, or jelly). This mixture should be swallowed and not chewed. The entire mixture must be swallowed to ensure that the child received the entire dose.

Special Instructions

May cause dizziness in some people. Until it is known how the child will react to the medicine, activities that require mental alertness (such as physical education and playground activity) should be restricted.

For older children, dry mouth may be relieved by chewing gum or sucking on hard candy or ice chips. Younger children may need extra liquids.

N o t e s

Spironolactone S

Common Uses

Spironolactone belongs to the class of medicines called diuretics. Spironolactone is used to treat hypertension and to remove excess body fluid caused by certain diseases because it increases the volume of urine eliminated from the body.

Usual Doses

Children: 1.0–3.5 mg/kg/day divided into equal doses given every 6–24 hours. Maximum dose 200 mg/day.

Adults: 25–200 mg/day divided into equal doses given every 6–24 hours. Maximum dose 200 mg/day.

Medication Interactions

Spironolactone may increase the risk for the development of adverse side effects of:

potassium acetate	potassium citrate
potassium acid	potassium gluconate
potassium bicarbonate	potassium iodide
potassium chloride	potassium phosphate

Adverse Side Effects

Minor: Nausea, diarrhea, vomiting, headache, dizziness, drowsiness, dry mouth, rash, restlessness.

Severe: Confusion; breast enlargement; fever; hair growth; muscle cramps or weakness; fatigue; numbness or tingling in the hands, lips, or feet; awareness of heartbeat; unusual or irregular heartbeat; stomach cramps; uncontrolled movements; clumsiness; anxiety; difficulty breathing; unusual sweating; rash; joint pain or swelling; deepened voice.

Brand Name

Aldactone
(tablet)

S

Storage and Administration

The oral medicine should be stored in a cool, dry place away from light. Prolonged exposure to heat, moisture, or light can damage the medicine.

It is best to take spironolactone with food or milk to increase the amount of medicine that the body absorbs and to help prevent upset stomach.

If the child is unable to swallow the tablet, it can be crushed and mixed with water or soft food (such as applesauce, pudding, jam, or jelly). This mixture should be swallowed and not chewed. The entire mixture must be swallowed to ensure that the child received the full dose.

Special Instructions

May cause dizziness or drowsiness in some people. Until it is known how the child will react to the medicine, activities that require mental alertness (such as physical education and playground activity) should be restricted.

May cause dizziness upon standing; therefore, always have the child stand up slowly. If the child becomes dizzy, she should be instructed to sit or lie down immediately.

For older children, dry mouth may be relieved by chewing gum or sucking on hard candy or ice chips. Younger children may need extra liquids.

N o t e s

Sucralfate S

Common Uses

Sucralfate is used to treat stomach ulcers, because it binds to the ulcer and prevents stomach acid from hurting it.

Usual Dose

Children: 40–80 mg/kg/day divided into equal doses given every 6 hours.

Adults: 1 g/dose given 2–4 times a day.

Medication Interactions

Sucralfate may decrease the effectiveness of:

ciprofloxacin   ofloxacin

lomefloxacin   phenytoin

norfloxacin

Adverse Side Effects

Minor: Nausea, constipation, diarrhea, upset stomach, back pain, dizziness, drowsiness, dry mouth.

Severe: Rash, itching, sweating.

Storage and Administration

The oral medicine should be stored in a cool, dry place away from light. Prolonged exposure to heat, moisture, or light can damage the medicine.

Before each dose is measured, the liquid form of sucralfate should be shaken well. The liquid may be stored at room temperature and does not need to be refrigerated.

Sucralfate should be given 1 hour before a meal and at bedtime.

Do not allow the child to take antacids within 1 hour before or 1 hour after taking sucralfate.

Brand Name
Carafate (tablet, liquid)

S

If the child is not able to swallow the tablet, place the whole tablet in a small amount of water until softened and then have him drink it. Crushing the tablet is not necessary.

Special Instructions

May cause drowsiness or dizziness in some people. Until it is known how the child will react to the medicine, activities that require mental alertness (such as physical education and playground activity) should be restricted.

For older children, dry mouth may be relieved by chewing gum or sucking on hard candy or ice chips. Younger children may need extra liquids.

The child's physician should be notified as soon as possible if he throws up and the vomit contains blood or looks like coffee grounds, or if he passes black or bloody stools.

N o t e s

Sulfamethoxazole S

Common Uses

Sulfamethoxazole belongs to the class of medicines called antibiotics, which are used to treat a variety of bacterial infections. Sulfamethoxazole is prescribed for infections of the middle ear, urinary tract, and respiratory tract, because it prevents the bacteria from growing.

Sulfamethoxazole is effective only against bacterial infections, not those caused by viruses, parasites, or yeast.

Usual Dose

Infants older than 2 months and Children: 50–60 mg/kg/day divided into equal doses given every 12 hours. Maximum dose 75 mg/kg/day or 3 g/day.

Adults: 1–2 g/day divided into equal doses given every 8–12 hours.

Medication Interactions

Sulfamethoxazole may increase the risk for the development of adverse side effects of:

acetohexamide   tolazamide

chlorpropamide   tolbutamide

glipizide

Sulfamethoxazole may decrease the effectiveness of:

cyclosporine

Adverse Side Effects

Minor: Nausea, vomiting, diarrhea, loss of appetite, headache, dizziness, weakness, fatigue, increased sensitivity to sunlight.

Severe: Rash; sore throat; fever; difficulty swallowing; mouth sores; swelling of the neck; painful urination; blood in the urine; numbness, burning, or tingling in the hands or feet; joint pain or aching; lower back pain; unusual bruising or bleeding; yellow skin or eyes.

Brand Names

Gantanol
  (tablet, liquid)
Urobak
  (tablet)

S

Storage and Administration

The oral medicine should be stored in a cool, dry place away from light. Prolonged exposure to heat, moisture, or light can damage the medicine.

Before the dose is measured, the liquid form of sulfamethoxazole should be shaken well. The liquid may be stored at room temperature and does not need to be refrigerated.

The child should take this medicine with a full glass of water and drink plenty of water between doses.

Sulfamethoxazole works best when taken on an empty stomach (1 hour before a meal or 2–3 hours after a meal).

If the child is unable to swallow the tablet, it can be crushed and mixed with water. This mixture should be swallowed and not chewed. The entire mixture must be swallowed to ensure that the child received the full dose.

Special Instructions

Notify the child's physician if the infection worsens or does not improve within 3–5 days.

May cause dizziness in some children. Until it is known how the child will react to the medicine, activities that require mental alertness (such as physical education and playground activity) should be restricted.

Have the child avoid prolonged exposure to sunlight because this medication causes her to be more sensitive to it.

N o t e s

Sulfisoxazole S

Common Uses

Sulfisoxazole belongs to the class of medicines called antibiotics, which are used to treat a variety of bacterial infections. Sulfisoxazole is prescribed for infections of the middle ear, urinary tract, and pelvic inflammatory disease, because it prevents the bacteria from growing.

Sulfisoxazole is effective only against bacterial infections, not those caused by viruses, parasites, or yeast.

Brand Name

Gantrisin
(tablet, liquid)

Usual Dose

Infants older than 2 months and Children: 120–150 mg/kg/day divided into equal doses given every 4–6 hours. Maximum dose 6 g/day.

Adults: 4–8 g/day divided into equal doses given every 4–6 hours.

Medication Interactions

Sulfisoxazole may increase the risk for the development of adverse side effects of:

acetohexamide	tolazamide
chlorpropamide	tolbutamide
glipizide	

Sulfisoxazole may decrease the effectiveness of:

cyclosporine

Adverse Side Effects

Minor: Headache, nausea, diarrhea, dizziness, weakness, fatigue, increased sensitivity to sunlight, discolored urine (black, brown, or yellowish-brown).

Severe: Rash; sore throat; fever; aching joints and muscles; yellow skin or eyes; numbness, tingling or burning feeling in the hands or feet; blood in the urine; painful urination; difficulty swallowing; low back pain; neck swelling; unusual bruising or bleeding.

S

Storage and Administration

The oral medicine should be stored in a cool, dry place away from light. Prolonged exposure to heat, moisture, or light can damage the medicine.

Before the dose is measured, the liquid form of sulfisoxazole should be shaken well. The liquid may be stored at room temperature and does not need to be refrigerated.

Have the child take this medicine with a full glass of water and drink plenty of water between doses.

Sulfisoxazole works best when taken on an empty stomach (1 hour before a meal or 2–3 hours after a meal).

If the child is unable to swallow the tablet, it can be crushed and mixed with water. This mixture should be swallowed and not chewed. The entire mixture must be swallowed to ensure that the child received the full dose.

Special Instructions

Notify the child's physician if the infection worsens or does not improve within 3–5 days.

May cause the urine to become black, brown, or yellowish-brown in color. This effect is harmless.

Have the child avoid prolonged exposure to sunlight, because sulfisoxazole causes him to be more sensitive to it.

May cause dizziness in some children. Until it is known how the child will react to the medicine, activities that require mental alertness (such as physical education and playground activity) should be restricted.

N o t e s

Terbutaline sulfate

T

Common Uses

Terbutaline sulfate belongs to the class of medicines called bronchodilators. Terbutaline sulfate is used to treat and prevent asthma attacks and to improve breathing difficulties caused by various other non–infection-related respiratory problems. Terbutaline sulfate opens the airways and prevents them from closing again.

Usual Dose

TABLET

Children younger than 12 years: 0.05 mg/kg/dose given every 8 hours. Maximum dose 0.15 mg/kg/dose or 5 mg/day.

Children 12–15 years old: 2.5 mg/dose given every 8 hours. Maximum dose 7.5 mg/day.

Children older than 15 years and Adults: 2.5–5 mg/dose given every 8 hours. Maximum dose 15 mg/day.

ORAL INHALATION

See the Medication Administration section for instructions on the proper use of an oral inhaler (page 10).

Children older than 12 years and Adults: 2 puffs every 4–6 hours.

Medication Interactions

No major medication interactions have been found with other oral medications.

Adverse Side Effects

Minor

ORAL INHALATION: Dry throat and mouth. The side effects listed under the Tablet and Syrup section also can occur when too many inhalations are given or when the medicine is given too often.

TABLET AND SYRUP: Nervousness, headache, fast heartbeat, trembling, insomnia, increased blood pressure, dizziness, upset stomach, nausea, vomiting, hyperactivity, flushing.

Brand Names

Brethaire
(tablet,
oral inhaler)

Brethine
(tablet)

Bricanyl
(tablet)

T

Severe: Chest pain, hallucinations, difficult or painful urination, rash, irregular heartbeat.

Storage and Administration

The oral medicine should be stored in a cool, dry place away from light. Prolonged exposure to heat, moisture, or light can damage the medicine.

The inhaler should be kept in a cool place. Do not puncture or expose the inhaler to prolonged periods of heat.

If upset stomach occurs, terbutaline can be given with food or milk.

If the child is unable to swallow the tablet, it can be crushed and mixed with water or soft food (such as applesauce, pudding, jam, or jelly). This mixture should be swallowed and not chewed. The entire mixture must be swallowed to ensure that the child received the full dose.

For proper use of the inhaler read the medication administration section entitled Oral Inhaler.

To prevent dry throat and mouth, have the child rinse her mouth with water after each inhalation.

If the child is receiving more than 1 puff of the oral inhaler, give the second puff at least 1 minute after the first one.

If the child is receiving another inhaled medicine for asthma, the entire inhaled terbutaline dose should be given at least 10–15 minutes before the other inhaled medicine is given, or as directed by a physician.

Special Instructions

Consult the child's physician about giving extra inhalations, because increasing the number of inhalations may be dangerous.

Children may be more susceptible to side effects of insomnia, nervousness, hyperactivity, and fast heartbeat than adults.

Have the child avoid eating excessive amounts of chocolate and drinking beverages containing caffeine, because they may make the child susceptible to insomnia, irritability, and hyperactivity.

May cause dizziness in some children. Until it is known how the child will react to the medicine, activities that require mental alertness (such as physical education and playground activity) should be restricted.

For older children, dry mouth may be relieved by chewing gum or sucking on hard candy or ice chips. Younger children may need extra liquids.

Terfenadine

T

Common Uses

Terfenadine belongs to the class of medicines called antihistamines. Terfenadine is used to treat runny and stuffy noses and sneezing caused by allergies, because it blocks the chemical histamine, which causes the allergic reaction.

Usual Dose

Children 3–6 years old: 15 mg/dose given twice a day.

Children 7–12 years old: 30 mg/dose given twice a day.

Children older than 12 years and Adults: 60 mg/dose given twice a day.

Medication Interactions

Medications that may increase the risk for the development of terfenadine adverse side effects are:

azithromycin

clarithromycin

erythromycin base

erythromycin estolate

erythromycin ethylsuccinate

erythromycin stearate

erythromycin with sulfisoxazole

fluconazole

itraconazole

ketoconazole

troleandomycin

Adverse Side Effects

Minor: Headache; fatigue; drowsiness; dizziness; dry mouth, nose, and throat; weakness; insomnia; nausea.

Severe: Muscle or bone pain, numbness or tingling of the hands or feet, sore throat, fever, difficulty breathing, irregular heartbeat, yellow skin or eyes, nosebleeds.

T

Storage and Administration

The oral medicine should be stored in a cool, dry place away from light. Prolonged exposure to heat, moisture, or light can damage the medicine.

Terfenadine works best when taken on an empty stomach (1 hour before a meal or 2–3 hours after a meal), but if upset stomach occurs it can be given with food or milk.

If the child is unable to swallow the tablet, it can be crushed and mixed with a small amount of water or soft food (such as applesauce, pudding, jam, or jelly). This mixture should be swallowed and not chewed. The entire mixture must be swallowed to ensure that the child received the full dose.

Special Instructions

May cause drowsiness and dizziness in some people. Until it is known how the child will react to the medicine, activities that require mental alertness (such as physical education and playground activity) should be restricted.

For older children, dry mouth may be relieved by chewing gum or sucking on hard candy or ice chips. Younger children may need extra liquids.

N o t e s

Tetracycline hydrochloride T

Common Uses

Tetracycline belongs to the class of medicines called antibiotics, which are used to treat a variety of bacterial infections. Tetracycline is prescribed for infections of the eye, mouth, and female genitalia. Tetracycline also can be used to treat acne (bacteria is partially responsible for acne lesions) and Lyme disease. Tetracycline is able to treat these infections because it prevents the bacteria from growing.

Tetracycline is effective only against bacterial infections, not those caused by viruses, parasites, or yeast.

Usual Dose

TABLET, CAPSULE, AND LIQUID

Children older than 8 years: 25–50 mg/kg/day divided into equal doses given every 6 hours.

Adults: 1–2 g/day divided into equal doses given every 6–12 hours.

SKIN SOLUTION AND OINTMENT

Children: No dosages have been determined, but the adult doses may be prescribed.

Adults: Apply as directed to the infected area 2 times a day.

EYE OINTMENT AND SUSPENSION

See the Medication Administration section for instructions on the proper application of eye ointment and drops (page 8).

Children and Adults

EYE OINTMENT: Apply a small amount as directed every 2–12 hours.

EYE SUSPENSION: Apply 1–2 drops in each infected eye 2–4 times a day.

Brand Names

Achromycin
(eye ointment,
eye suspen-
sion, skin
ointment)
Achromycin V
(capsule,
liquid)
Nor-Tet
(capsule)
Panmycin
(capsule)
Sumycin
(tablet,
capsule,
liquid)
Tetracap
(capsule)
Tetralan
(capsule,
liquid)
Tetram
(capsule)
Topicycline
(skin solution)

T

Medication Interactions

Medications that may decrease the effectiveness of tetracycline are:

antacids	penicillin G
amoxicillin	penicillin V
ampicillin	potassium citrate
bismuth salts	sodium acetate
cloxacillin	sodium bicarbonate
dicloxacillin	sodium citrate
iron salts	sodium lactate
nafcillin	zinc gluconate
oxacillin	zinc sulfate

Tetracycline increases the risk for the development of adverse side effects of:

digoxin

Adverse Side Effects

Minor

ORAL MEDICINE: Nausea, diarrhea, upset stomach, vomiting, increased sensitivity to sunlight, tooth discoloration in children who do not yet have their permanent teeth.

SKIN MEDICINE: Dry skin, mild burning or stinging sensation, itching, mild redness of skin, skin discoloration.

EYE MEDICINE: Blurred vision, mild burning or stinging.

Severe: Difficulty breathing, joint pain, rash, hives, skin blistering, sore throat, fever, yellow skin or eyes, persistent burning or stinging of the eyes or skin.

Storage and Administration

The oral medicine should be stored in a cool, dry place away from light. Prolonged exposure to heat, moisture, or light can damage the medicine.

The skin solution and ointment, eye ointment, and suspension may be stored at room temperature.

Before the dose is measured, the liquid form of tetracycline should be shaken well. The liquid may be stored at room temperature and does not need to be refrigerated. After receiving the liquid medicine from the pharmacy, it is good only for 14 days; therefore, always check the expiration date on the prescription label before using.

Tetracycline works best when taken on an empty stomach (1 hour before a meal or 2–3 hours after a meal).

The child should take this medicine with a full glass of water.

If the child is unable to swallow pills, the tablets can be crushed or the capsules opened and mixed with a small amount of water. The entire mixture must be swallowed to ensure that the child received the full dose.

Do not allow the child to drink milk or eat ice cream, cottage cheese, cheese, or other dairy products 2 hours before or 2 hours after taking tetracycline.

Do not allow the child to take antacids within 2 hours before or 2 hours after taking tetracycline.

Special Instructions

The child's physician should be notified if the infection worsens or does not improve within 3–5 days.

Have the child avoid prolonged exposure to sunlight, because this medication causes him to be more sensitive to it.

Tetracycline can cause irreversible tooth discoloration in children who do not yet have all their permanent teeth.

T

Skin solution is to be used only on the skin; be careful not to get it into the child's eyes.

The skin medicine may cause the child's skin to become yellowish in color. This effect is harmless and the discoloration usually can be removed with water.

N o t e s

Theophylline T

Common Uses

Theophylline belongs to the class of medicines called bronchodilators. Theophylline is used to prevent and treat asthma attacks and various other non–infection-related respiratory problems, because it opens up the airways, making it easier to breathe.

Usual Dose

The dosing intervals given below are for the non–long-acting medicine. The long-acting medicine may be given to children older than 1 year of age. When the long-acting medicine is given to these children, the dosing interval is every 8–12 hours.

Children 6 weeks–12 months old: Dosage may be calculated based on the child's weight or age.

Dose based on child's weight:

Children 6 weeks–6 months old: 6–15 mg/kg/day divided into equal doses given every 6–8 hours.

Children 6–12 months old: 12–22 mg/kg/day divided into equal doses given every 6–8 hours.

Dose based on the child's age:

$(0.2 \times$ age in weeks$) + 5 =$ dose in mg/kg/day.

or

$(0.3 \times$ age in weeks$) + 8 =$ dose in mg/kg/day.

Children 1–9 years old: 20–24 mg/kg/day divided into equal doses given every 4–6 hours.

Children 9–12 years old: 16 mg/kg/day divided into equal doses given every 4–6 hours.

Children 12–16 years old

Nonsmokers: 13 mg/kg/day divided into equal doses given every 4–6 hours.

Smokers: 16 mg/kg/day divided into equal doses given every 4–6 hours.

Brand Names

Aerolate
  (long-acting
  capsule,
  liquid)
Aerolate JR
  (long-acting
  capsule)
Aerolate SR
  (long-acting
  capsule)
Aquaphyllin
  (liquid)
Bronkodyl
  (capsule)
Elixophyllin
  (capsule,
  liquid)
Elixophyllin SR
  (long-acting
  capsule)
Lanophyllin
  (liquid)
Slo-bid
  Gyrocaps
  (long-acting
  capsule)
Slo-Phyllin
  (tablet, liquid)
Slo-Phyllin
  Gyrocaps
  (long-acting
  capsule)

(continued next page)

T

Brand Names

(continued)

Theo-24
  (long-acting
  capsule)
Theobid
  Duracaps
  (long-acting
  capsule)
Theobid Jr.
  Duracaps
  (long-acting
  capsule)
Theoclear-80
  (liquid)
Theoclear L.A.
  (long-acting
  capsule)
Theo-Dur
  (long-acting
  tablet)
Theo-Dur
  Sprinkle
  (long-acting
  capsule)
Theolair
  (tablet, liquid)
Theolair-SR
  (long-acting
  tablet)

Children older than 16 years and Adults

NONSMOKERS: 10 mg/kg/day divided into equal doses given every 4–6 hours. Maximum dose 900 mg/day.

SMOKERS: 16 mg/kg/day divided into equal doses given every 4–6 hours.

Medication Interactions

Medications that may increase the risk for the development of theophylline adverse side effects are:

cimetidine	erythromycin with sulfisoxazole
ciprofloxacin	
disulfiram	mexiletine
enoxacin	norfloxacin
erythromycin base	propranolol
erythromycin estolate	thiabendazole
erythromycin ethylsuccinate	ticlopidine
	troleandomycin
erythromycin stearate	

Medications that may decrease the effectiveness of theophylline are:

carteolol	phenytoin
dextrothyroxine*	pindolol
levothyroxine*	primidone
liothyronine*	propranolol
liotrix*	propylthiouracil*
methimazole*	rifampin
penbutolol	thyroid*
phenobarbital	timolol

*The occurrence of the interactions depends on how well the thyroid disease is controlled and if the medications were started before or after the theophylline.

Theophylline may decrease the effectiveness of:

phenytoin

Adverse Side Effects

Minor: Nausea, vomiting, upset stomach, stomach pain, diarrhea, headache, trembling, nervousness, insomnia, dizziness, fast heartbeat.

Severe: Black or tarry stools, seizures, difficulty breathing, rash, severe stomach pain, irregular heartbeat.

Storage and Administration

The oral medicine should be stored in a cool, dry place away from light. Prolonged exposure to heat, moisture, or light can damage the medicine.

The liquid may be stored at room temperature and does not need to be refrigerated.

Theophylline tablets and capsules should be taken with a full glass of water.

Theophylline works best when taken on an empty stomach (1 hour before a meal or 2–3 hours after a meal), but if upset stomach occurs the liquid or non–long-acting dosage forms can be given with food unless otherwise instructed by the child's physician.

Some of the long-acting and non–long-acting capsules or tablets can be opened or crushed and sprinkled onto soft food (such as applesauce, pudding, jam, or jelly). This mixture should be swallowed and not chewed. The entire mixture must be swallowed to ensure that the child received the full dose.

Special Instructions

Have the child avoid eating excessive amounts of chocolate or drinking products that contain caffeine, because caffeine-related side effects (headache, trembling, nervousness, insomnia, fast heartbeat) are more likely to occur.

May cause dizziness in some people. Until it is known how the child will react to the medicine, activities that require mental alertness (such as physical education and playground activity) should be restricted.

The child's physician should be notified as soon as possible if black or tarry stools occur.

T hioridazine hydrochloride

Brand Names

Mellaril
(tablet, con-
centrate)
Mellaril-S
(liquid)
Thioridazine
HCl
(tablet,
concentrate)
Thioridazine
HCl Intensol
(concentrate)

Common Uses

Thioridazine belongs to the class of medicines called tranquilizers. Thioridazine is used to treat various forms of mental illness and agitation, because it blocks chemicals responsible for imbalanced nerve transmissions in the brain.

Usual Dose

Children 2–12 years old: 0.5–3 mg/kg/day divided into equal doses given 2–3 times a day.

Children 12 years or older and Adults: 25–100 mg/dose given 3 times a day. Maximum dose 800 mg/day.

Medication Interactions

Medications that may increase the risk for the development of thioridazine adverse side effects are:

alcohol   propranolol

atropine   scopolamine

benztropine   trihexyphenidyl

oxybutynin

Thioridazine may decrease the effectiveness of:

guanethidine

Medications that may increase the risk of sedation, drowsiness, and dizziness when combined with thioridazine are:

brompheniramine

chlorpheniramine

diphenhydramine

Adverse Side Effects

Minor: Dry mouth, constipation, dizziness, drowsiness, stuffy nose, restlessness, pink or reddish-brown urine, increased sensitivity to sunlight.

Severe: Chest pain; seizures; difficulty swallowing or breathing; fever; sore throat; rash; stomach pain; yellow skin or eyes; unusual bruising or bleeding; blurred vision; trembling; twitching; drooling; unintentional movements of the face, mouth, or tongue.

Storage and Administration

The oral medicine should be stored in a cool, dry place away from light. Prolonged exposure to heat, moisture, or light can damage the medicine.

Before the dose is measured, the liquid form of thioridazine should be shaken well. The liquid and concentrate may be stored at room temperature and do not need to be refrigerated.

If the child is unable to swallow the tablet, it can be crushed and mixed with water, fruit juice, or soft food (such as applesauce, pudding, jam, or jelly). This mixture should be swallowed and not chewed. The entire mixture must be swallowed to ensure that the child received the entire dose.

Exposure to sunlight will damage the concentrate.

If upset stomach occurs, thioridazine can be given with food or milk.

Avoid touching the concentrate or having it touch the child's skin because an itchy rash may occur. If the concentrate does come into contact with the skin, rinse the skin thoroughly with water.

The concentrate should be mixed with half a cup or more of orange juice, grapefruit juice, lemonade, or water. Prepare the mixture just before giving the dose. The medicine will be damaged if left in the mixture; therefore, do not premix and store.

Special Instructions

May cause drowsiness and dizziness in some people. Until it is known how the child will react to the medicine, activities that require mental alertness (such as physical education and playground activity) should be restricted.

May cause dizziness upon standing; therefore, always have the child stand up slowly. If the child becomes dizzy, she should be instructed to sit or lie down immediately.

Limit the child's play on hot days because thioridazine increases the risk of heat stroke.

For older children, dry mouth may be relieved by chewing gum or sucking on hard candy or ice chips. Younger children may need extra liquids.

T

May cause the urine to become pink to reddish-brown in color. This effect is harmless.

In children with a seizure disorder, this medicine may cause seizures even if child's condition is currently controlled.

Have the child avoid prolonged exposure to sunlight, because thioridazine may cause her to be more sensitive to it.

Do not abruptly stop giving the child the medication unless directed to by the physician. Suddenly stopping the medicine can cause nausea, vomiting, upset stomach, headache, increased heart rate, or trembling.

Notes

Thiothixene T

Common Uses

Thiothixene belongs to the class of medicines called tranquilizers. Thiothixene is used to treat various forms of mental illness and agitation, because it blocks chemicals responsible for imbalanced nerve transmissions in the brain.

Usual Dose

Children younger than 12 years: 0.25 mg/kg/day given in divided doses. Dosing guidelines in this age group have not been well established.

Children 12 years or older and Adults: Start with 2 mg/dose given 3 times a day and increase the dose according to the physician's directions. Maximum dose 60 mg/day.

Medication Interactions

No major medication interactions have been found with other oral medications.

Adverse Side Effects

Minor: Dry mouth, constipation, dizziness, drowsiness, stuffy nose, restlessness, pink to reddish-brown urine, increased sensitivity to sunlight.

Severe: Chest pain; seizures; difficulty swallowing or breathing; fever; sore throat; rash; stomach pain; yellow skin or eyes; unusual bruising or bleeding; blurred vision; trembling; twitching; drooling; unintentional movements of the face, mouth, and tongue.

Storage and Administration

The oral medicine should be stored in a cool, dry place away from light. Prolonged exposure to heat, moisture, or light can damage the medicine.

Brand Name

Navane
(capsule,
concentrate)

T

The concentrate may be stored at room temperature and does not need to be refrigerated.

Keep the concentrate out of sunlight because this will damage the medicine.

If upset stomach occurs, thiothixene can be given with food or milk.

Avoid touching the concentrate or having it touch the child's skin because an itchy rash may occur. If the concentrate does come into contact with the skin, rinse the skin thoroughly with water.

The concentrate should be mixed with half a cup or more of apple or orange juice, grapefruit juice, milk, water, or with a small amount of soft food (such as applesauce, pudding, jam, or jelly). Prepare the mixture just before giving the dose. The medicine will be damaged if left in the mixture; therefore, do not premix and store.

If the child is unable to swallow the capsule, it can be opened and mixed with water or soft food (such as applesauce, pudding, jam, or jelly). This mixture should be swallowed and not chewed. The entire mixture must be swallowed to ensure that the child received the full dose.

Special Instructions

May cause drowsiness and dizziness in some people. Until it is known how the child will react to the medicine, activities that require mental alertness (such as physical education and playground activity) should be restricted.

May cause dizziness upon standing; therefore, always have the child stand up slowly. If the child becomes dizzy, he should be instructed to sit or lie down immediately.

Limit the child's playing on hot days, because thiothixene increases the risk of heat stroke.

For older children, dry mouth may be relieved by chewing gum or sucking on hard candy or ice chips. Younger children may need extra liquids.

May cause the urine to become pink to reddish-brown in color; this is harmless.

In children with a seizure disorder, this medicine may cause seizures even if the child's condition is currently controlled.

T

Have the child avoid prolonged exposure to sunlight, because this medication may cause him to be more sensitive to it.

Do not abruptly stop this medicine. Suddenly stopping it may cause nausea, vomiting, upset stomach, headache, increased heart rate, or trembling.

Notes

Trazodone hydrochloride

Brand Name

Desyrel
(tablet)

Common Uses

Trazodone belongs to the class of medicines called antidepressants. Trazodone is used to treat people with various forms of depression, because it increases the concentration of chemicals in the brain that help counteract the depression.

Usual Dose

Children 6–18 years old: 1.5–2 mg/kg/day divided into equal doses given 3 times a day. Maximum dose 6 mg/kg/day.

Adults: 150 mg/day divided into equal doses given 3 times a day. Maximum dose 600 mg/day.

Medication Interactions

No major medication interactions have been found with other oral medications.

Adverse Side Effects

Minor: Nausea, vomiting, heartburn, diarrhea, constipation, dizziness, drowsiness, blurred vision, dry mouth, bad taste in the mouth, headache, nervousness, increased sensitivity to sunlight.

Severe: Tight chest, chest pain, difficulty breathing, difficult or painful urination, blood in the urine, nightmares, hallucinations, confusion, loss of coordination, tingling of the fingers or toes, unusual or fast heartbeat, awareness of heartbeat, trembling, unusual excitement, rash, ringing in the ears, unusual bruising or bleeding, unusual fatigue or weakness, fainting.

Storage and Administration

The oral medicine should be stored in a cool, dry place away from light. Prolonged exposure to heat, moisture, or light can damage the medicine.

It is best to give trazodone with food to prevent upset stomach, decrease dizziness associated with the medicine, and increase the amount of medicine taken into the body.

Do not crush the tablet because the powder tastes bad. If necessary, the tablet can be crushed and mixed with water or soft food (such as applesauce, pudding, jam, or jelly). This mixture should be swallowed and not chewed. The entire mixture must be swallowed to ensure that the child received the full dose.

Special Instructions

May cause drowsiness or dizziness in some people. Until it is known how the child will react to the medicine, activities that require mental alertness (such as physical education and playground activity) should be restricted.

May cause dizziness upon standing; therefore, always have the child stand up slowly. If the child becomes dizzy, she should be instructed to sit or lie down immediately.

For older children, dry mouth may be relieved by chewing gum or sucking on hard candy or ice chips. Younger children may need extra liquids.

Have the child avoid prolonged exposure to sunlight because trazodone causes her to be more sensitive to it.

Do not abruptly stop this medicine. Suddenly stopping the medicine can cause nausea, headache, or upset stomach.

N o t e s

T riamcinolone

Brand Names

Aristocort
(tablet,
skin ointment,
skin cream)

Aristocort A
(skin ointment,
skin cream)

Atolone
(tablet)

Azmacort
(oral inhaler)

Delta-Tritex
(skin ointment,
skin cream)

Flutex
(skin ointment,
skin cream)

Kenacort
(tablet, liquid)

Kenalog
(skin ointment,
skin cream,
skin lotion)

Kenalog-H
(skin cream)

Kenonel
(skin cream)

Nasacort
(nasal inhaler)

Triacet
(skin cream)

Triderm
(skin cream)

Common Uses

Triamcinolone belongs to the class of medicines called corticosteroids. Oral inhalation of the medicine is used to treat asthma. Nasal inhalation is used to provide relief of stuffy nose and nasal irritation and discomfort due to hay fever and allergies. Oral tablets and liquids are used to treat asthma, allergies, inflammatory diseases, and various other problems. Skin ointment, creams, and lotions are used to relieve the itching, redness, and discomfort of various skin diseases and rashes caused by poison oak and poison ivy. Triamcinolone affects many different substances in the body that may cause or worsen these conditions.

Usual Dose

ORAL INHALATION

See the Medication Administration section for instructions on the proper use of an oral inhaler (page 10).

Children 6–12 years old: 1–2 inhalations 3–4 times a day. Maximum dose 12 inhalations/day.

Children older than 12 years and Adults: 2 inhalations 3–4 times a day. Maximum dose 16 inhalations/day.

NASAL INHALATION

See the Medication Administration section for instructions on the proper use of a nasal inhaler (page 16).

Children older than 12 years and Adults: Start with 2 sprays in each nostril once a day and increase the dose according to the physician's directions. Maximum dose 4 sprays in each nostril/day.

TABLET AND LIQUID

Children older than 12 years and Adults: 4–100 mg/day divided into equal doses given 1–4 times a day.

SKIN OINTMENT, CREAM, AND LOTION

Children and Adults: Apply as directed to the infected area 2–4 times a day.

Medication Interactions

A medication that may increase the risk for the development of triamcinolone adverse side effects is:

troleandomycin

Medications that may decrease the effectiveness of triamcinolone are:

phenobarbital   primidone

phenytoin   rifampin

Triamcinolone decreases the effectiveness of:

aspirin   magnesium salicylate

bismuth subsalicylate   salsalate

choline salicylate   sodium salicylate

Adverse Side Effects

Minor

ORAL INHALATION: Yeast growth in the mouth, hoarseness, dry mouth, cough, bad taste in the mouth, headache, dizziness.

NASAL INHALATION: Irritation and burning of nose, sneezing, yeast growth in the nose, headache, stuffy or runny nose, bad taste in the mouth, dizziness.

TABLET OR LIQUID: Round face, weight gain, acne, upset stomach, nausea, vomiting, increased appetite, dizziness.

SKIN MEDICINE: Acne, dry skin, mild burning or stinging sensation, itching, minor rash.

Severe: Rash, hives, skin blistering, loss of skin color, skin infection at the site where the medicine is used, difficulty swallowing, increased thirst, headache, seizures, insomnia, fatigue, abnormal hair growth, black or tarry stools, sore throat, fever, hallucinations, irregular heartbeat, blurred vision, stomach pain, nightmares, difficulty breathing, unusual weakness, leg cramps.

Storage and Administration

The oral medicine should be stored in a cool, dry place away from light. Prolonged exposure to heat, moisture, or light can damage the medicine.

T

The liquid may be stored at room temperature and does not need to be refrigerated.

The skin ointment, cream, and lotion may be stored at room temperature.

The inhaler should be kept in a cool place. Do not puncture or expose the inhaler to prolonged periods of heat.

For proper use of the oral and nasal inhaler read the appropriate medication administration section.

After oral inhalation, have the child rinse his mouth with water. This helps prevent some of the side effects associated with oral inhalation.

If the child is also taking an orally inhaled bronchodilator (such as albuterol, metaproterenol, or terbutaline) give the entire bronchodilator dose at least 10–15 minutes, or as directed by a physician, before giving triamcinolone oral inhalations.

If the child is unable to swallow the tablet, it can be crushed and mixed with water, fruit juice, carbonated beverages, or soft food (such as applesauce, pudding, jam, or jelly). This mixture should be swallowed and not chewed. The entire mixture must be swallowed to ensure that the child received the entire dose.

It is best to give triamcinolone with food or milk to decrease or prevent upset stomach.

Special Instructions

Oral inhalation of triamcinolone is used to prevent asthma attacks, but it cannot treat an asthma attack. When an asthma attack occurs this medicine will not help.

May cause dizziness in some people. Until it is known how the child will react to the medicine, activities that require mental alertness (such as physical education and playground activity) should be restricted.

If the child has been taking this medicine for more than 1 week, do not allow him to abruptly stop taking it. Suddenly stopping the oral medicine (tablet and liquid) can cause nausea, vomiting, weakness, fever, shortness of breath, stomach or back pain, or dizziness.

If the child has been taking triamcinolone for more than 1 week, notify the physician who prescribed the triamcinolone if a serious injury or illness occurs.

Skin ointment, cream, and lotion are to be used only on the skin; be careful not to get it into the child's eyes.

Do not use tight-fitting diapers when using the skin medicine in the diaper area.

The child's physician should be notified as soon as possible if black or tarry stools occur.

Trifluoperazine hydrochloride

Common Uses

Trifluoperazine belongs to the class of medicines called tranquilizers. Trifluoperazine is used to treat various forms of mental illness and agitation, because it blocks the chemical responsible for imbalanced nerve transmissions in the brain.

Usual Dose

Children 6–12 years old: 1 mg/day divided into equal doses given 1–2 times a day. Maximum dose 15 mg/day.

Children older than 12 years and Adults: 5–10 mg/day divided into equal doses given 1–2 times a day. Maximum dose 40 mg/day.

Medication Interactions

Medications that may increase the risk for the development of trifluoperazine adverse side effects are:

alcohol	oxybutynin
atropine	scopolamine
benztropine	trihexyphenidyl

Trifluoperazine may decrease the effectiveness of:

guanethidine

Medications that may increase the risk of sedation, drowsiness, and dizziness when combined with trifluoperazine are:

brompheniramine

chlorpheniramine

diphenhydramine

Brand Name

Stelazine
(tablet,
concentrate)

T

Adverse Side Effects

Minor: Dry mouth, constipation, dizziness, drowsiness, stuffy nose, restlessness, pink to reddish-brown urine, increased sensitivity to sunlight.

Severe: Chest pain; seizures; difficulty swallowing or breathing; fever; sore throat; rash; stomach pain; yellow skin or eyes; unusual bruising or bleeding; blurred vision; trembling; twitching; drooling; unintentional movements of the face, mouth, and tongue.

Storage and Administration

The oral medicine should be stored in a cool, dry place away from light. Prolonged exposure to heat, moisture, or light can damage the medicine.

The concentrate may be stored at room temperature and does not need to be refrigerated.

Keep the concentrate out of sunlight because this will damage the medicine.

If upset stomach occurs, trifluoperazine can be given with food or milk.

Avoid touching the concentrate or having it touch the child's skin because an itchy rash may occur. If the concentrate does come into contact with the skin, rinse the skin thoroughly with water.

The concentrate should be mixed with half a cup or more of orange juice, grapefruit juice, pineapple juice, apricot juice, milk, water, or carbonated beverage, or with a small amount of soft food (such as applesauce, pudding, jam, or jelly). Prepare the mixture just before giving the dose. The medicine will be damaged if left in the mixture; therefore, do not premix and store.

If the child is unable to swallow the tablet, it can be crushed and mixed with a small amount of water or soft food (such as applesauce, pudding, jam, or jelly). This mixture should be swallowed and not chewed. The entire mixture must be swallowed to ensure that the child received the full dose.

Special Instructions

May cause sedation, drowsiness, and dizziness in some people. Until it is known how the child will react to the medicine, activities that require mental alertness (such as physical education and playground activity) should be restricted.

May cause dizziness upon standing; therefore, always have the child stand up slowly. If the child becomes dizzy, she should be instructed to sit or lie down immediately.

Limit the child's playing on hot days, because trifluoperazine increases the risk of heat stroke.

For older children, dry mouth may be relieved by chewing gum or sucking on hard candy or ice chips. Younger children may need extra liquids.

May cause the urine to become pink to reddish-brown in color; this effect is harmless.

In children with a seizure disorder, trifluoperazine may cause seizures even if the child's condition is currently controlled.

Do not abruptly stop this medicine. Suddenly stopping it may cause nausea, vomiting, upset stomach, headache, increased heart rate, or trembling.

Have the child avoid prolonged exposure to sunlight, because this medication may cause her to be more sensitive to it.

Notes

Trimethoprim with Sulfamethoxazole

Brand Names

Bactrim
  (tablet, liquid)
Bactrim DS
  (tablet)
Cotrim
  (tablet)
Cotrim D.S.
  (tablet)
Cotrim
  Pediatric
  (liquid)
Septra
  (tablet, liquid)
Septra DS
  (tablet)
TMP-SMZ
  (tablet)

Common Uses

Trimethoprim with Sulfamethoxazole (sometimes called co-trimoxazole) belongs to the class of medicines called antibiotics. This medicine combination contains 1 part of trimethoprim and 5 parts of sulfamethoxazole. Antibiotics are used to treat a variety of bacterial infections. Trimethoprim with sulfamethoxazole is prescribed for infections of the middle ear, urinary tract, and respiratory tract, because it prevents the bacteria from growing. This medication also can be used to prevent infection.

Trimethoprim with sulfamethoxazole is effective only against bacterial infections, not those caused by viruses, parasites, or yeast.

Usual Dose

TREATMENT OF INFECTION

Children: 6-12 mg/kg/day of trimethoprim divided into equal doses given every 12 hours.

Adults: 1 double strength (DS) tablet given every 12 hours.

PREVENTION OF INFECTION

Children: 2 mg/kg of trimethoprim given once daily.

Adults: 1 single-strength (SS) or 1 double-strength (DS) tablet given once daily.

Medication Interactions

A medication that may increase the risk for the development of trimethoprim with sulfamethoxazole adverse side effects is:

dapsone

Trimethoprim with sulfamethoxazole may increase the risk for the development of adverse side effects of:

cyclosporine   phenytoin

dapsone   warfarin

Adverse Side Effects

Minor: Headache, nausea, diarrhea, dizziness, weakness, fatigue, increased sensitivity to sunlight, sore mouth or tongue, unusual taste in the mouth.

Severe: Rash, sore throat, fever, aching joints or muscles, yellow skin or eyes, numbness, tingling or burning feeling in the hands or feet, blood in the urine, unusual bruising or bleeding, difficulty breathing or swallowing, painful urination, low back pain, neck swelling, swollen or inflamed tongue.

Storage and Administration

The oral medicine should be stored in a cool, dry place away from light. Prolonged exposure to heat, moisture, or light can damage the medicine.

Before the dose is measured, the liquid form of trimethoprim with sulfamethoxazole should be shaken well. The liquid may be stored at room temperature and does not need to be refrigerated.

If the child is unable to swallow the tablet, it can be crushed and mixed with water. The entire mixture must be swallowed to ensure that the child received the entire dose.

Have the child take this medicine with a full glass of water and drink plenty of water in between doses.

Should be taken on an empty stomach (1 hour before a meal or 2–3 hours after a meal).

Special Instructions

The child's physician should be notified if the infection worsens or does not improve within 3–5 days.

Have the child avoid prolonged exposure to sunlight, because this medication may cause him to be more sensitive to it.

May cause drowsiness or dizziness in some children. Until it is known how the child will react to the medicine, activities that require mental alertness (such as physical education and playground activity) should be restricted.

Valproic acid

Brand Name

**Depakene
(capsule,
liquid)**

Common Uses

Valproic acid belongs to the class of medicines called anticonvulsants. Valproic acid is used to treat and control seizures, because it increases the concentration of chemicals that help prevent the spread of the seizure throughout the brain.

Usual Dose

Children and Adults: 10–60 mg/kg/day divided into equal doses given 1–3 times a day.

Medication Interactions

Medications that may increase the risk for the development of valproic acid adverse side effects are:

aspirin	magnesium salicylate
bismuth subsalicylate	salsalate
choline salicylate	sodium salicylate

Medications that may decrease the effectiveness of valproic acid are:

carbamazepine

phenytoin

Valproic acid increases the risk for the development of adverse side effects of:

carbamazepine	phenytoin
phenobarbital	primidone

Adverse Side Effects

Minor: Nausea, vomiting, diarrhea, upset stomach, dizziness, drowsiness, trembling, headache, constipation.

Severe: Unusual bruising or bleeding, rash, yellow skin or eyes, blurred or double vision, unusual eye movements, swelling of the feet and legs, weakness, stomach pain.

V

Storage and Administration

The oral medicine should be stored in a cool, dry place away from light. Prolonged exposure to heat, moisture, or light can damage the medicine.

The liquid may be stored at room temperature and does not need to be refrigerated.

If upset stomach occurs, valproic acid can be given with food.

The capsule should be swallowed whole with a full glass of water. Do not open the capsule because the contents may cause mouth and throat irritation.

The liquid should be diluted in half a glass of water or milk. Prepare the mixture just before giving the dose. The medicine will be damaged if left in the mixture; therefore, do not premix and store.

Special Instructions

May cause drowsiness and dizziness in some people. Until it is known how the child will react to the medicine, activities that require mental alertness (such as physical education and playground activity) should be restricted.

Do not suddenly stop giving valproic acid to the child unless instructed to do so by a physician. Suddenly stopping this medication may cause severe seizures to occur.

Notes

W arfarin sodium

Brand Names

Coumadin
(tablet)
Panwarfin
(tablet)
Sofarin
(tablet)

Common Uses

Warfarin belongs to the class of medicines called anticoagulants. Warfarin is used to prevent the formation of blood clots; it blocks the production of certain blood-clotting substances.

Usual Dose

Infants and Children: 0.05–0.34 mg/kg/dose given once a day.

Adults: 2–15 mg/dose given once a day.

Medication Interactions

Medications that may decrease the effectiveness of warfarin are:

aprobarbital	phenobarbital
carbamazepine	primidone
cholestyramine	propylthiouracil*
glutethimide	rifabutin
griseofulvin	rifampin
levothyroxine*	secobarbital
liothyronine*	thyroid*
liotrix*	vitamin K
methimazole*	

*These interactions depend on how well the thyroid disease is controlled and whether the child began taking the medication before or after warfarin was begun.

Warfarin may increase the risk for the development of adverse side effects of:

phenytoin

W

Medications that may increase the risk of stomach bleeding when combined with warfarin are:

diclofenac	ketorolac
fenoprofen	naproxen
ibuprofen	piroxicam
indomethacin	sulindac
ketoprofen	tolmentin

Medications that may increase the risk of bleeding when combined with warfarin are:

amiodarone	metronidazole
aspirin	miconazole
chloral hydrate	nalidixic acid
cimetidine	oxandrolone
clofibrate	oxymetholone
danazol	oxyphenbutazone
dextrothyroxine	phenylbutazone
dipyridamole	phenytoin
disulfiram	propylthiouracil
erythromycin base	quinidine
erythromycin estolate	quinine
erythromycin ethylsuccinate	stanozolol
erythromycin stearate	sulfamethizole
fluconazole	sulfamethoxazole
fluoxymesterone	sulfisoxazole
levothyroxine	sulfinpyrazone
liothyronine	thyroid
liotrix	trimethoprim with sulfamethoxazole
methimazole	

methyl salicylate

methyltestosterone

vitamin E

Adverse Side Effects

Minor: Nausea, vomiting, stomach cramps, decreased appetite, diarrhea, blurred vision, red-orange urine.

Severe: Blood in the urine, stool, saliva, or vomit; vomit that looks like coffee-grounds; nosebleeds, continuous bleeding from small cuts; unusual or severe bruising or bleeding; purple-black skin; rash; fever; stomach pain; joint swelling; burning sensation in the feet; muscle or back pain, headache; weakness; fatigue; difficult or painful urination; dizziness; yellow skin or eyes.

Storage and Administration

The oral medicine should be stored in a cool, dry place away from light. Prolonged exposure to heat, moisture, or light can damage warfarin.

Should be taken on an empty stomach (1 hour before a meal or 2–3 hours after a meal).

If the child is unable to swallow the tablet, it can be crushed and mixed with water or juice. The entire mixture must be swallowed to ensure that the child received the full dose.

Special Instructions

Do not allow the child to take aspirin or aspirin-containing medicine while taking warfarin unless directed by a physician.

While the child is taking warfarin, acetaminophen should be the only medicine used for pain or fever. Avoid using any medicine that is a nonsteroidal antiinflammatory drug (NSAID) (such as ibuprofen and naproxen), unless directed by a physician.

Warfarin may cause the urine to become red-orange in color; this effect is harmless.

Have the child avoid all contact sports while taking this medicine.

The child's physician should be notified as soon as possible if vomiting that looks like coffee grounds or has blood in it, or black or bloody stools occur.

Zalcitabine Z

Common Uses

Zalcitabine belongs to the class of medicines called antivirals. Different antivirals are able to treat different viral infections. Zalcitabine is prescribed for children infected with HIV, the virus that causes AIDS, because it prevents the virus from growing.

Zalcitabine is effective only against HIV infections, not those caused by other viruses, bacteria, parasites, or yeast.

Usual Dose

Children who weigh more than 30 kg (66 lb) and Adults: In combination with zidovudine: 2.25 mg/day divided into equal doses given every 8 hours.

Medication Interactions

Medications that may increase the risk for the development of zalcitabine adverse side effects are:

chloramphenicol	metronidazole
dapsone	nitrofurantoin
hydralazine	phenytoin
isoniazid	zidovudine

Adverse Side Effects

Minor: Fever, joint pain, mouth sores.

Severe: Nausea; vomiting; stomach pain; numbness, tingling, or pain in the fingers or toes; decreased amount of urine.

Storage and Administration

The oral medicine should be stored in a cool, dry place away from light. Prolonged exposure to heat, moisture, or light can damage the medicine.

Brand Name

Hivid
(tablet)

Z

Should be taken on an empty stomach (1 hour before a meal or 2–3 hours after a meal).

If the child is unable to swallow the tablet, it can be crushed and mixed with water. The entire mixture must be swallowed to ensure that the child received the entire dose.

Special Instructions

Report any vomiting; stomach pain; or numbness, tingling, or pain in the hands or feet to the child's physician immediately.

N o t e s

Zidovudine Z

Common Uses

Zidovudine (sometimes called azidothymidine) belongs to the class of medicines called antivirals. Different antivirals are able to treat different viral infections. Zidovudine is prescribed for children infected with HIV, the virus that causes AIDS, because it prevents the virus from growing.

Zidovudine is effective only against HIV infections, not those caused by other viruses, bacteria, parasites, or yeast.

Usual Dose

Children 3 months–12 years old: 90–180 mg/m²/dose given every 6 hours. Maximum dose 200 mg/dose.

Children older than 12 years and Adults

NO SYMPTOMS OF THE DISEASE: 100 mg/dose given every 4 hours while awake.

SYMPTOMS OF THE DISEASE: 200 mg/dose given every 4 hours for 1 month, then 100 mg/dose given every 4 hours.

Medication Interactions

A medication that may increase the risk for the development of zidovudine adverse side effects is:

zalcitabine

A medication that may cause rash, feeling of being unwell, muscle pain, or fever when combined with zidovudine is:

probenecid

Adverse Side Effects

Minor: Nausea, diarrhea, dizziness, headache, insomnia, loss of appetite, muscle soreness, bluish-brown colored hands or nails.

Brand Name
Retrovir (capsule, liquid)

Z

Severe: Chills, difficulty breathing, lip or tongue swelling, pale skin, fever, stomach pain, sore throat, fatigue, seizures, muscle weakness.

Storage and Administration

The oral medicine should be stored in a cool, dry place away from light. Prolonged exposure to heat, moisture, or light can damage the medicine.

The liquid may be stored at room temperature and does not need to be refrigerated.

Zidovudine should be given 30 minutes before or 1 hour after a meal, but if upset stomach occurs, it can be given with food.

If the child is unable to swallow the capsule, it can be opened and mixed with water or a small amount of soft food (such as applesauce, pudding, jam, or jelly). This mixture should be swallowed and not chewed. The entire mixture must be swallowed to ensure that the child received the full dose.

Special Instructions

May cause dizziness in some children. Until it is known how the child will react to the medicine, activities that require mental alertness (such as physical education and playground activity) should be restricted.

N o t e s

BIBLIOGRAPHY

1. **American Academy of Pediatric Committee on Drugs.** *Transfer of drugs and other chemicals into human milk.* Pediatrics 1994;93:137-50.

2. **Benitz WE, Tatro DS.** *The pediatric drug handbook.* 2nd ed. Chicago: Year Book Medical Publishers, 1988.

3. **Briggs GG, Freeman RK, Yaffe SJ.** *Drugs in pregnancy and lactation.* 3rd ed. Baltimore: Williams and Wilkins, 1990.

4. **Griffith HW.** *Complete guide to prescription and non-prescription drugs.* New York: Putnam Publishing Group, 1995.

5. **Johnson KB.** *The Harriet Lane Handbook: a manual for pediatric house officers.* 13th ed.. St. Louis: Mosby-Year Book, 1993.

6. **Knoben JE, Anderson PO, eds.** *Handbook of clinical drug data.* 7th ed. Hamilton, IL: Drug Intelligence Publications, 1993.

7. **Lacey C, Armstrong LL, Lipsy RJ, Lance LL.** *Drug information handbook.* 2nd ed. Hudson, OH: Lexi-comp, 1994-1995.

8. **Loeb S, Hamilton HK, eds.** *Photoguide to drug administration.* Springhouse, PA: Springhouse Corp., 1992.

9. **Long JW, Rybacki JJ.** *The essential guide to prescription drugs.* New York: HarperPerennial Publishers, 1995.

10. **McEvoy GK, ed.** *AHFS drug information.* Bethesda, MD: American Society of Hospital Pharmacists, 1994.

11. **Olin BR, ed.** *Facts and comparisons: loose-leaf drug information service.* St. Louis: Facts and Comparisons, updated monthly.

12. **Pagliaro LA, Pagliaro AM.** *Problems in pediatric drug therapy.* 3rd ed. Hamilton, IL: Drug Intelligence Publications, 1995.

13. *Physicians' desk reference.* 48th ed. Montvale, NJ: Medical Economics, 1994.

14. *Prescription drugs.* Lincolnwood, IL: Publications International, 1992.

15. **Shannon MT, Wilson BA.** *Govoni and Hayes drugs and nursing implications.* 7th ed. East Norwalk, CT: Appleton and Lange, 1992.

16. **Silverman HM, Chilnick LD, eds.** *The pill book.* 5th ed. New York: Bantam Books, 1992.

17. **Smith DL.** *Understanding prescription drugs.* New York: Pocket Books, 1987.

18. **Taketomo CK, Hodding JH, Kraus DM.** *Pediatric dosage handbook.* 2nd ed. Hudson, OH: Lexi-comp, Inc., 1993-1994.

19. **Tatro DS, ed.** *Drug interaction facts.* St. Louis: Facts and Comparisons, updated quarterly.

INDEX

*There is information on these medications (listed by generic name) in the section on Medications and Breast Feeding (page 28).

Index

Index

Index

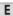

Index

Ery-Tab,* see *Erythromycin base, 165*
Erythrocin Stearate,* see
  Erythromycin stearate, 171
Erythromycin base,* *165*
Erythromycin estolate,* *167*
Erythromycin ethylsuccinate,* *169*
Erythromycin stearate,* *171*
Erythromycin with Sulfisoxazole,
  173
Eryzol, see *Erythromycin with Sulfi-
  soxazole, 173*
Esidrix,* see *Hydrochlorothiazide, 202*
Eskalith,* see *Lithium, 28*
Eskalith CR,* see *Lithium, 28*
Espotabs,* see *Phenolphthalein, 31*
Estrace,* see *Estradiol, 30*
Estraderm,* see *Estradiol, 30*
Estradiol,* *30*
Ethambutol,* *175*
Ethosuximide,* *177*
Evac-U-Gen,* see *Phenolphthalein, 31*
Excedrin IB,* see *Ibuprofen, 207*
Ex-Lax,* see *Phenolphthalein, 31*

F, G, H

Famotidine,* *30*
Feen-a-mint,* see *Phenolphthalein,
  31*
Felbamate, *179*
Felbatol, see *Felbamate, 179*
Feldene,* see *Piroxicam, 31*
Feosol, see *Ferrous sulfate, 183*
Feratab, see *Ferrous sulfate, 183*
Fergon, see *Ferrous gluconate, 181*
Fer-In-Sol, see *Ferrous sulfate, 183*
Ferndex, see *Dextroamphetamine, 142*
Fero-Gradumet Filmtab, see
  Ferrous sulfate, 183
Ferospace, see *Ferrous sulfate, 183*
Ferralet, see *Ferrous gluconate, 181*
Ferralet Slow Release, see *Ferrous
  gluconate, 181*
Ferralyn Lanacaps, see *Ferrous sulfate,
  183*
Ferra-TD, see *Ferrous sulfate, 183*
Ferrous gluconate, *181*
Ferrous sulfate, *183*
Flagyl,* see *Metronidazole, 237*
Flecainide,* *30*
Floxin,* see *Ofloxacin, 29*
Fluconazole, *185*

Flumadine, see *Rimantadine hydro-
  chloride, 297*
Flunisolide, *187*
Fluoride,* *30*
Fluoritab,* see *Fluoride, 30*
Fluoxetine hydrochloride,* *189*
Flura,* see *Fluoride, 30*
Flura-Drops,* see *Fluoride, 30*
Flura-Loz,* see *Fluoride, 30*
Flurbiprofen,* *30*
Flutex, see *Triamcinolone, 326*
Folic acid,* *30*
Formula Q,* see *Quinine sulfate, 31*
Furadantin,* see *Nitrofurantoin, 248*
Furalan,* see *Nitrofurantoin, 248*
Furanite,* see *Nitrofurantoin, 248*
Furosemide,* *191*
Gabapentin, *193*
Gantanol, see *Sulfamethoxazole, 303*
Gantrisin,* see *Sulfisoxazole, 305*
Gastrocrom, see *Cromolyn sodium, 128*
Genahist, see *Diphenhydramine
  hydrochloride, 154*
Genaphed,* see *Pseudoephedrine
  hydrochloride, 287*
Genprin,* see *Aspirin, 29*
Ginseng,* *29*
Glyate, see *Guaifenesin, 195*
Guaifenesin, *195*
Guiatuss, see *Guaifenesin, 195*
G-well,* see *Lindane, 226*
Haldol,* see *Haloperidol, 197*
Halofed,* see *Pseudoephedrine
  hydrochloride, 287*
Haloperidol,* *197*
Halotussin, see *Guaifenesin, 195*
1% HC, see *Hydrocortisone, 204*
Heroin,* *28*
Hexadrol, see *Dexamethasone, 137*
Hismanal, see *Astemizole, 70*
Hivid, see *Zalcitabine, 339*
Hold DM, see *Dextromethorphan, 144*
Humibid L.A., see *Guaifenesin, 195*
Humibid Sprinkle, see *Guaifenesin, 195*
Humulin 70/30,* see *Insulin, 215*
Humulin L,* see *Insulin, 215*
Humulin N,* see *Insulin, 215*
Humulin R,* see *Insulin, 215*
Hycort, see *Hydrocortisone, 204*
Hydralazine hydrochloride,* *200*
Hydramine, see *Diphenhydramine
  hydrochloride, 154*

Index

Hydrochlorothiazide,* 202
Hydrocortisone, 204
HydroDIURIL,* see
Hydrochlorothiazide, 202
Hydro-Par,* see Hydrochlorothiazide, 204
HydroTex, see Hydrocortisone, 204
Hydroxychloroquine sulfate,* 30
Hygroton,* see Chlorthalidone, 30
Hytone, see Hydrocortisone, 204
Hytuss, see Guaifenesin, 195
Hytuss 2X, see Guaifenesin, 195

I, J, K

Ibuprin,* see Ibuprofen, 207
Ibuprofen,* 207
Ilosone,* see Erythromycin estolate, 167
Ilozyme, see Pancrelipase, 256
Imipramine hydrochloride,* 210
Imodium,* see Loperamide, 30
Imodium A-D,* see Loperamide, 30
Imodium A-D Caplets,* see
Loperamide, 30
Inderal,* see Propranolol hydrochloride, 283
Inderal LA,* see Propranolol hydrochloride, 283
Indocin,* see Indomethacin, 213
Indocin SR,* see Indomethacin, 213
Indomethacin,* 213
Indomethacin SR,* see Indomethacin, 213
Insulin,* 215
Intal, see Cromolyn sodium, 128
Iodine,* 29
Iodo-Niacin,* see Iodine, 29
Isoniazid,* 217
Isoptin,* see Verapamil, 31
Isoptin SR,* see Verapamil, 31
Istizin,* see Danthron, 30
Janimine,* see Imipramine hydrochloride, 210
Junior Strength Feverall,* see Acetaminophen, 48
Kanamycin,* 30
Kantrex,* see Kanamycin, 30
Kaopectate II Caplets,* see Loperamide, 30
Karidium,* see Fluoride, 30
Keflet,* see Cephalexin, 30
Keflex,* see Cephalexin, 30
Keftab,* see Cephalexin, 30

Kenacort, see Triamcinolone, 326
Kenalog, see Triamcinolone, 326
Kenalog-H, see Triamcinolone, 326
Kenonel, see Triamcinolone, 326
Ketoconazole, 220
Ketorolac,* 30
Klonopin,* see Clonazepam, 20
Kondremul Plain,* see Mineral oil, 30
Ku-Zyme, see Pancrelipase, 256
Kwell,* see Lindane, 226

L, M

Labetalol,* 29
Laniazid,* see Isoniazid, 217
Laniazid C.T.,* see Isoniazid, 217
Lanophyllin,* see Theophylline, 315
Lanoxicaps,* see Digoxin, 151
Lanoxin,* see Digoxin, 151
Lasix,* see Furosemide, 191
Lax Pills,* see Phenolphthalein, 31
Laxative Pills,* see Phenolphthalein, 31
Lead,* 29
Ledercillin VK,* see Penicillin V potassium, 262
Legatrin,* see Quinine sulfate, 31
Lente Insulin,* see Insulin, 215
Levonorgestrel,* 30
Levothroid, see Levothyroxine sodium, 224
Levothyroxine sodium, 224
Levoxine, see Levothyroxine sodium, 224
Lincocin,* see Lincomycin, 29
Lincomycin,* 29
Lindane,* 226
Lioresal,* see Baclofen, 30
Liquid Pred,* see Prednisone, 275
Lithane,* see Lithium, 28
Lithium,* 28
Lithobid,* see Lithium, 28
Lithonate,* see Lithium, 28
Lithotabs,* see Lithium, 28
Lomefloxacin,* 29
Loniten,* see Minoxidil, 30
Loperamide,* 30
Lopressor,* see Metoprolol, 29
Lorabid, see Loracarbef, 228
Loracarbef, 228
Lorazepam,* 29
Lotrimin, see Clotrimazole, 122
Lotrimin AF, see Clotrimazole, 122
Lugol's Solution,* see Iodine, 29

Index

Luride Lozi-Tabs,* see *Fluoride, 30*
M-KYA,* see *Quinine sulfate, 31*
Macrodantin,* see *Nitrofurantoin, 248*
Magnaprin,* see *Aspirin, 29*
Magnesium hydroxide,* *30*
Marijuana,* *28*
Maxaquin,* see *Lomefloxacin, 29*
Maxidex, see *Dexamethasone, 137*
Medihaler-Epi, see *Epinephrine, 163*
Medilax,* see *Phenolphthalein, 31*
Medipren,* see *Ibuprofen, 207*
Medroxyprogesterone,* *30*
Mefenamic acid,* *30*
Mellaril, see *Thioridazine hydrochloride, 318*
Mellaril S, see *Thioridazine hydrochloride, 318*
Mephyton,* see *Phytonadione, 31*
Mesoridazine,* *29*
Mestinon,* see *Pyridostigmine, 31*
Mestranol,* *30*
Metaprel, see *Metaproterenol sulfate, 230*
Metaproterenol sulfate, *230*
Methadone,* *29*
Methadone Intensol,* see *Methadone, 29*
Methergine,* see *Methylergonovine, 29*
Methimazole,* *30*
Methocarbamol,* *30*
Methotrexate,* *28*
Methyldopa,* *30*
Methylergonovine,* *29*
Methylphenidate hydrochloride, *233*
Methyprylon,* *30*
Meticorten,* see *Prednisone, 275*
Metoclopramide,* *235*
Metoprolol,* *29*
MetroGel,* see *Metronidazole, 237*
Metronidazole,* *237*
Mexiletine,* *30*
Mexitil,* see *Mexiletine, 30*
Midol 200,* see *Ibuprofen, 207*
Milk of Magnesia,* see *Magnesium hydroxide, 30*
Milkinol,* see *Mineral oil, 30*
Mineral oil,* *30*
Minocin,* see *Minocycline hydrochloride, 240*
Minocycline hydrochloride,* *240*
Minoxidil,* *30*

Mol-Iron, see *Ferrous sulfate, 183*
Morphine,* *29*
Motilium,* see *Domperidone, 30*
Motrin IB,* see *Ibuprofen, 207*
MS Contin,* see *Morphine, 29*
MSIR,* see *Morphine, 29*
Myambutol,* see *Ethambutol, 175*
Mycelex, see *Clotrimazole, 122*
Mycostatin, see *Nystatin, 250*
Mycostatin Pastilles, see *Nystatin, 250*
Myidyl,* see *Triprolidine, 31*
Myotonachol, see *Bethanechol chloride, 80*
Mysoline,* see *Primidone, 277*
Mytussin, see *Guaifenesin, 195*

N, O

Nadolol,* *29*
Nafcillin sodium, *242*
Nalidixic acid,* *31*
Naprosyn,* see *Naproxen, 244*
Naproxen,* *244*
Nasacort, see *Triamcinolone, 326*
Nasalcrom, see *Cromolyn sodium, 128*
Nasalide, see *Flunisolide, 187*
Naturetin,* see *Bendroflumethiazide, 30*
Navane, see *Thiothixene, 321*
NegGram,* see *Nalidixic acid, 31*
Nembutal,* see *Pentobarbital, 29*
Neo-mercazole,* see *Carbimazole, 30*
Neopap,* see *Acetaminophen, 48*
Nestrex,* see *Pyridoxine, 31*
Neurontin, see *Gabapentin, 193*
Nicotine* (smoking), *28*
Nifedipine,* *246*
Nilstat, see *Nystatin, 250*
Nitrofan,* see *Nitrofurantoin, 248*
Nitrofurantoin,* *248*
Nix, see *Permethrin, 264*
Nizatidine,* *31*
Nizoral, see *Ketoconazole, 220*
Noctec,* see *Chloral hydrate, 29*
NoDoz,* see *Caffeine, 30*
Noludar,* see *Methyprylon, 30*
Norethynodrel,* *31*
Norfloxacin,* *29*
Normodyne,* see *Labetalol, 29*
Noroxin,* see *Norfloxacin, 29*
Norpace,* see *Disopyramide, 30*
Norpace CR,* see *Disopyramide, 30*
Norplant,* see *Levonorgestrel, 30*

Index

Index

Index

Index

Index

American Association of
Poison Control Centers
Certified Regional Poison Centers, April 1995

ALABAMA

Alabama Poison Center, Tuscaloosa
408-A Paul Bryant Drive
Tuscaloosa, AL 35401
Emergency Phone 205/345-0600 or
  800/462-0800 (AL only)

Regional Poison Control Center
The Children's Hospital of Alabama
1600 7th Ave. South
Birmingham, AL 35233-1711
Emergency Phone 205/939-9201, 205/933-4050, or
  800/292-6678 (AL only)

ARIZONA

Arizona Poison and Drug Information Center
Arizona Health Sciences Center, Rm. #3204-K
1501 N. Campbell Ave.
Tucson, AZ 85724
Emergency Phone: 602/626-6016 or
  800/362-0101 (AZ only)

Samaritan Regional Poison Center
Good Samaritan Regional Medical Center
Ancillary-1
1111 E. McDowell Road
Phoenix, AZ 85006
Emergency Phone: 602/253-3334

CALIFORNIA

**Central California Regional Poison
  Control Center**
Valley Children's Hospital
3151 N. Millbrook, IN31
Fresno, CA 93703
Emergency Phone: 209/445-1222 or
  800/346-5922 (Central CA only)

San Diego Regional Poison Center
UCSD Medical Center
200 West Arbor Drive
San Diego, CA 92103-8925
Emergency Phone: 619/543-6000 or
  800/876-4766 (in 619 area code only)

**San Francisco Bay Area Regional Poison
  Control Center**
San Francisco General Hospital
1001 Potrero Ave., Building 80, Room 230
San Francisco, CA 94110
Emergency Phone: 800/523-2222

Santa Clara Valley Regional Poison Center
Valley Health Center, Suite 310
750 South Bascom Ave.
San Jose, CA 95128
Emergency Phone: 408/885-6000 or
  800/662-9886 (CA only)

**University of California, Davis,
  Medical Center Regional Poison
  Control Center**
2315 Stockton Blvd.
Sacramento, CA 95817
Emergency Phone: 916/734-3692 or
  800/342-9293 (Northern CA only)

COLORADO

Rocky Mountain Poison and Drug Center
645 Bannock St.
Denver, CO 80204
Emergency Phone: 303/629-1123

DISTRICT OF COLUMBIA

National Capital Poison Center
3201 New Mexico Avenue NW, Suite 310
Washington, DC 20016
Emergency Phone: 202/625-3333 or
  202/362-8563 (TTY)

FLORIDA

**Florida Poison Information Center–
  Jacksonville**
University Medical Center, University of Florida
  Health Science Center–Jacksonville
655 West 8th Street
Jacksonville, FL 32209
Emergency Phone: 904/549-4480 or
  800/282-3171 (FL only)

**The Florida Poison Information Center
  and Toxicology Resource Center**
Tampa General Hospital, PO Box 1289
Tampa, FL 33601
Emergency Phone 813/253-4444 (in Tampa) or
  800/282-3171 (FL only)

GEORGIA

Georgia Poison Center
Grady Memorial Hospital
80 Butler Street S.E.
PO Box 26066
Atlanta, GA 30335-3801
Emergency Phone: 404/616-9000 or
  800/282-5846 (GA only)

INDIANA

Indiana Poison Center
Methodist Hospital of Indiana
1701 N. Senate Blvd., PO Box 1367
Indianapolis, IN 46206-1367
Emergency Phone: 317/929-2323 or
  800/382-9097 (IN only)

KENTUCKY

Kentucky Regional Poison Center of Kosair Children's Hospital
PO Box 35070
Louisville, KY 40232-5070
Emergency Phone: 502/629-7275 or
800/722-5725 (KY only)

MARYLAND

Maryland Poison Center
20 N. Pine St.
Baltimore, MD 21201
Emergency Phone: 410/528-7701 or
800/492-2414 (MD only)

National Capital Poison Center (DC suburbs only)
3201 New Mexico Avenue NW, Suite 310
Washington, DC 20016
Emergency Phone: 202/625-3333 or
202/362-8563 (TTY)

MASSACHUSETTS

Massachusetts Poison Control System
300 Longwood Ave.
Boston, MA 02115
Emergency Phone: 617/232-2120 or
800/682-9211

MICHIGAN

Poison Control Center
Children's Hospital of Michigan
3901 Beaubien Blvd.
Detroit, MI 48201
Emergency Phone: 313/745-5711

MINNESOTA

Hennepin Regional Poison Center
Hennepin County Medical Center
701 Park Ave.
Minneapolis, MN 55415
Emergency Phone: 612/347-3141; Petline:
612/337-7387; TDD: 612/337-7474

Minnesota Regional Poison Center
St. Paul-Ramsey Medical Center
640 Jackson Street
St. Paul, MN 55101
Emergency Phone: 612/221-2113

MISSOURI

Cardinal Glennon Children's Hospital Regional Poison Center
1465 S. Grand Blvd.
St. Louis, MO 63104
Emergency Phone: 314/772-5200 or
800/366-8888

MONTANA

Rocky Mountain Poison and Drug Center
645 Bannock St.
Denver, Co 80204
Emergency Phone: 303/629-1123

NEBRASKA

The Poison Center
8301 Dodge St.
Omaha, NE 68114
Emergency Phone: 402/390-5555 (in Omaha) or
800/955-9119 (NE & WY only)

NEW JERSEY

New Jersey Poison Information and Education System
201 Lyons Ave.
Newark, NJ 07112
Emergency Phone: 800/962-1253

NEW MEXICO

New Mexico Poison and Drug Information Center
University of New Mexico
Albuquerque, NM 87131-1076
Emergency Phone: 505/843-2551 or
800/432-6866 (NM only)

NEW YORK

Hudson Valley Regional Poison Center
Phelps Memorial Hospital Center
701 North Broadway
North Tarrytown, NY 10591
Emergency Phone: 914/366-3030 or
800/336-6997

Long Island Regional Poison Control Center
Winthrop University Hospital
259 First Street
Mineola, NY 11501
Emergency Phone: 516/542-2323, -2324,
-2325, or -3813

New York City Poison Control Center
NYC Department of Health
455 First Ave., Room 123
New York, NY 10016
Emergency Phone: 212/340-4494 or
212/POISONS; TDD: 212/689-9014

NORTH CAROLINA

Carolinas Poison Center
1000 Blythe Blvd.
PO Box 32861
Charlotte, NC 28232-2861
Emergency Phone: 704/355-4000 or
800/84-TOXIN (800/848-6946)

OHIO

Central Ohio Poison Center
700 Children's Drive
Columbus, OH 43205-2696
Emergency Phone: 614/228-1323, 614/461-2012,
800/682-7625, or 614/228-2272 (TTY)

**Cincinnati Drug & Poison Information Center
and Regional Poison Control System**
231 Bethesda Ave., ML 144
Cincinnati, OH 45267-0144
Emergency Phone: 513/558-5111 or
800/872-5111 (OH only)

OREGON

Oregon Poison Center
Oregon Health Sciences University
3181 S.W. Sam Jackson Park Road
Portland, OR 97201
Emergency Phone: 503/494-8968 or
800/452-7165 (OR only)

PENNSYLVANIA

Central Pennsylvania Poison Center
University Hospital
Milton S Hershey Medical Center
Hershey, PA 17033
Emergency Phone: 800/521-6110

**The Poison Control Center serving the
Greater Philadelphia metropolitan area**
One Children's Center
Philadelphia, PA 19104-4303
Emergency Phone: 215/386-2100

Pittsburgh Poison Center
3705 Fifth Ave.
Pittsburgh, PA 15213
Emergency Phone: 412/681-6669

RHODE ISLAND

Rhode Island Poison Center
593 Eddy St.
Providence, RI 02903
Emergency Phone: 401/277-5727

TEXAS

North Texas Poison Center
5201 Harry Hines Blvd.
PO Box 35926
Dallas, TX 75235
Emergency Phone: 214/590-5000 or
Texas Watts 800/441-0040

Southeast Texas Poison Center
The University of Texas Medical Branch
Galveston, TX 77550-2780
Emergency Phone: 409/765-1420 or
713/654-1701 (in Houston)

UTAH

Utah Poison Control Center
410 Chipeta Way, Suite 230
Salt Lake City, UT 84108
Emergency Phone: 801/581-2151 or
800/456-7707 (UT only)

VIRGINIA

Blue Ridge Poison Center
Box 67
Blue Ridge Hospital
Charlottesville, VA 22901
Emergency Phone: 804/924-5543 or
800/451-1428

**National Capital Poison Center
(Northern VA only)**
3201 New Mexico Avenue NW, Suite 310
Washington, DC 20016
Emergency Numbers: 202/625-3333 or
202/362-8563 (TTY)

WEST VIRGINIA

West Virginia Poison Center
3110 MacCorkle Ave. S.E.
Charleston, WV 25304
Emergency Phone: 304/348-4211 or
800/642-3625 (WV only)

WYOMING

The Poison Center
8301 Dodge St.
Omaha, NE 68114
Emergency Phone: 402/390-5555 (in Omaha) or
800/955-9119 (NE & WY only)